PRAISE FOR BILLY SUNDAY MARS...

"Billy Sunday Mars is a master teacher who makes the work of exercise really fun." —Marin Independant Journal

"He has amazing physical grace with an immense knowledge of the body and a great sense of humor." —Lyn

"A grandmother of six, I am now able to move in ways that I haven't for twenty years. He is helping me get my flexible, dancing body back. And people are complimenting me about being in shape. I feel like a sexy woman again." —Kathy

THE EXPERIMENT

BECAUSE EVERY BOOK IS A TEST OF NEW IDEAS

FIT FOR LOVE

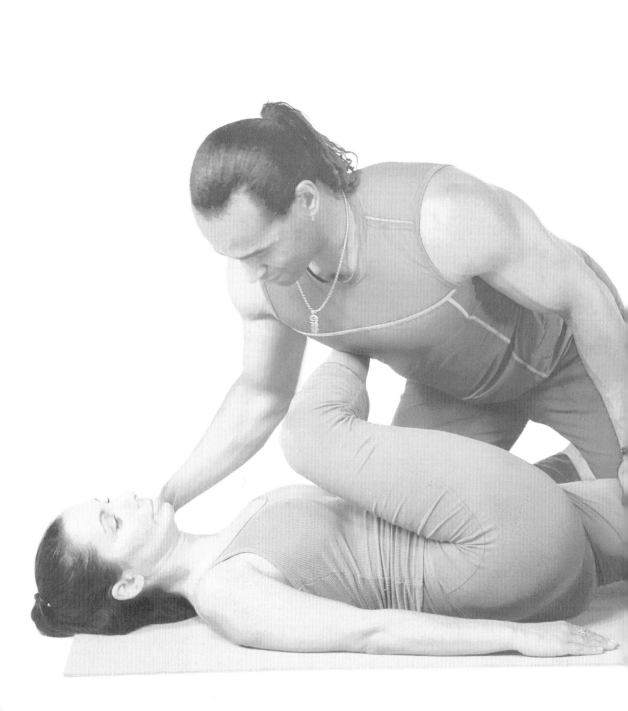

BILLY SUNDAY MARS

FIT FOR LOVE

Edited by Wendy Merrill

Photographs by Peter Ivory

Illustrations by Bonnie A. Neer

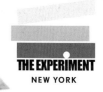

THE EXPERIMENT

NEW YORK

The Experiment, LLC
260 Fifth Avenue
New York, NY 10001-6425
www.theexperimentpublishing.com

Fit for Love includes stretches, exercises, and instructions for increasing sexual pleasure. The suggestions in this book are not intended as a substitute for consulting a professional trainer or health specialist. We strongly recommend that you check with your doctor before beginning a new workout routine. While care and caution were taken to give safe advice, readers should use personal judgment when applying the recommendations of this book. The author and publisher disclaim all liability in connection with the use of this book.

Library of Congress Control Number: 2009938390

ISBN 978-1-61519-009-6

COVER DESIGN BY HOWARD GROSSMAN | 12E DESIGN
COVER AND AUTHOR PHOTOGRAPHS BY PETER IVORY
TEXT DESIGN BY PAULINE NEUWIRTH, NEUWIRTH & ASSOCIATES, INC.

Manufactured in Canada
First published July 2010

10 9 8 7 6 5 4 3 2 1

CONTENTS

INTRODUCTION

*M*Y INTEREST IN pleasing women began in a tent made of blankets in my living room when I was ten years old. My sixteen-year-old sister Robyn always had her girlfriends over, and once, while they were waiting for Robyn to get ready, they asked if they could visit me in my tent. A bit scared, I agreed and invited them in. I remember being in awe of them—their shape, their smell, and the way they moved. They were different, very different. There wasn't much room in the tent, so we had to cuddle up and chat. I realized then that there was something surreal and superphysical about women, and that entertaining them should be an event.

My sisters' friends visited my tent regularly after that, and I brought them pillows and tea to encourage them to stay. As I got older I learned to cook, dance, sing, and play musical instruments. I started reading and writing poetry, and read of knights, chivalry, and troubadours. Eventually I discovered that there was an art to all of this. That art was to be found in the *Kama Sutra*.

Western culture has always been fascinated by the *Kama Sutra*, Tantra, and the "mysterious" sexual arts of the East. The *Kama Sutra* is an ancient Indian text that provides wonderful instruction on courtship, titillation, and exploring sexual positions. Tantra involves more rebellious rituals than common Buddhist practices: It focuses on elevating personal pleasure by prolonging coitus, increasing intimacy, and cultivating Kundalini (sexual energy), through and by increasing consciousness. Both teachings are considered paths to enlightenment, but what attracted me to them was the invitation to lose myself by pleasing another in the sensuality of a heightened erotic environment. Sex, understood in this way, is not an occurrence; it is an event. I, like many of you, longed to learn the "hidden secrets" of those arts that would make me a star in my own bedroom without having to become an acrobatic contortionist or yoga master. How could I create the deepest intimate connection with my partner? What were the best ways to achieve orgasm for my partner and myself? How did my anatomy affect how well I make love?

With experience, I realized that the problem with using the *Kama Sutra*, Tantra, or any other sensual guide as a road map to ecstasy was that it wouldn't work until I had prepared the vehicle—my body—for the journey. If you were taking your car on a long trip, would you just slide it in gear and drive without making sure it's ready for the road? All too often, sex is something we all "just do," with decidedly mixed results. Even my Tantra teachers, who had spent years teaching the sexual arts, were mindful of the many paths to pleasure but paid no attention to the vehicle that could get them there. I would try to imitate the positions in the books, but over time I realized that it was not the positions that were important, but how my lover and I *moved* when in those positions. If I was unable to move well enough to consistently stimulate my lover's internal areas, any and all books on sexual technique were useless. *The first purpose of this book is to help you learn how and why to condition your body to move in ways that feel wonderful to both you and your lover.*

My training is based on a process of isolating, improving, and integrating movements of the glute, groin, and pelvic muscles. One myth of the fitness industry is that you can't work or move the lower abdominals (abs) independent of the upper abs. As such, most aerobic and gym core-building exercises are repetitious and robotic, treating the abs like a single sheet of muscles. This philosophy of movement, unfortunately, often plays out in the bedroom. As a dancer, auto mechanic, student of the sexual arts, and subsequently as a trainer, I have studied how the human body works and have developed a fun and productive way to both isolate and train these muscles in my "Fit for Love" classes. I have turned the so-called "mystery" of the Eastern sexual arts into easy-to-master movements. Now I want to help you take these simple techniques from my classroom to your bedroom.

Let's face it: Every guy likes to think they're good at lovemaking, myself included. And because I was an erotic dancer when I was younger, there was no shortage of opportunities to find out. In dating a few of the women I met in the club, most of them older, I learned that I didn't move as well in bed as I did on the stage— not because the moves weren't good, but because they didn't apply horizontally. One night in bed, when I was trying a position from the *Kama Sutra*, I was stopped mid-stroke when my partner asked, "Billy, do you know why you're putting what where?" And she proceeded to teach me female anatomy, inside and out. Gradually I learned how to take my time and get to know what goes on inside a woman, and not just physically; her thoughts, feelings, and spiritual life are a major part of every intimate encounter. It is not just where, but how and when to touch a woman that matters. I began to see that women are both a maze and amazing if you take the time to look, feel, and explore them. This is one reason why I've never had a one-night stand. I prefer a long-term relationship, because that is the only way to get deep into the mystery that is woman.

After that relationship ended, I became a sort of "lover undercover." I asked a million and one questions of the women in the club and kept a notebook close at hand. I wanted to learn what not only I but we as men were doing wrong. To many women, I found out, the bedroom is a yellow-tape crime scene, not because sex is bad but because we're bad at it. These women taught me that romance and intimacy are important both in and out of bed, and that both areas need passion, skill, and attention to detail.

What I hear often from men is that they like women who enjoy sex and are able to express their sexuality. A woman expressing herself sexually—both verbally and physically—tells us that we turn you on, too! Men, whether they admit it or not, want someone sweet on the streets but wild in the sheets. Letting us know you have an erotic side does not mean we think you're easy! It just makes us feel desired. Having said that, I do think it is important for women to make men wait a little while before becoming intimate. If a man isn't willing to wait, he just wants sex, not you.

Bottom line: Both men and women want to feel desirable. Making love can be a physical and spiritual expression of our deepest emotional and physical yearnings. The more skilled we can become at expressing ourselves sexually and emotionally, the more fulfilling and rewarding our intimate connections will become.

The practices in this book will help you rev up your love life with your partner, first by increasing the mobility in your hips and spine to allow you better access to each other's pleasure points. The stretches and exercises in the first part of this book will target all the muscle groups that support the spine and pelvis, which enable you to move well in all directions. We will then apply your increased agility to some dance and martial arts moves. Finally, we will explore how your new moves translate into techniques you can use in various sex positions, from the bed to the couch and beyond. With practice, the two of you will ultimately be able to enter incredible heart and mind spaces together.

So how do you prepare yourself to become a great lover? I can help you to identify and work the muscles your body uses to make that magic happen, but it's important to remember that being "fit for love" is not simply being fit for sex. *It is also about building character, confidence, and connection by practicing erotic integrity.* Just as in learning the true understandings in the martial arts you would not go out and fight just anyone, in truly becoming fit for love, you should not go out and f$%k just anyone. The point is to develop and deepen your skill and understanding of intimate relations through regular practice and sharing with a worthy counterpart. The purpose of these exercises is to deepen intimacy and to encourage and celebrate monogamy. I believe that once we understand sex at a deep level and find the right partner, promiscuity will appear developmentally restrictive. By conditioning your body through this practice, you will also condition your mind and open your heart.

At times in this book, especially when I'm talking about sex, it may sound as though I'm speaking exclusively to men. Needless to say, as a heterosexual man, I can only speak from my experience with women. But rest assured that the core-building stretches, exercises, and general philosophy of the "Fit for Love" program are unisex and can benefit both men and women, gay or straight. Please apply what works best for you and just have fun with it. As with anything in life, you will get out of this practice what you're willing to put into it. I respectfully and playfully invite you to join me on a journey that will strengthen your body, improve your lovemaking skills, and connect you more deeply with your partner and yourself, opening yourself up to a better love life—and a better life.

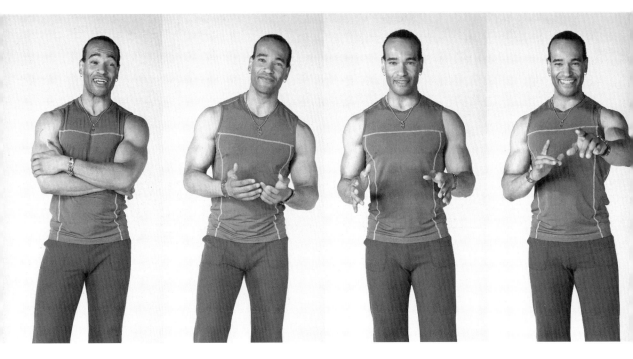

AS YOU GO through this book, please suspend judgment and just try to experience the moves—to improve rather than prove. After all is said and done, you and your lover will love the way you please each other.

FIT FOR LOVE

MEET YOUR HIPS AND SPINE

*L*ET'S FACE IT, folks: Stiff hips pose a big problem for lovemaking. Ask any woman for her two biggest complaints about men in bed and she'll tell you tight lips and stiff hips. If you have a problem puckering up or your stiff hips tucker you out, the only thing she'll want more than flowers to make up for it is batteries. Guys, if you're a dud instead of a stud, you're going to find yourself out-screwed by her Rabbit, because, frankly, there's almost no competing with ten thousand RPMs.

Many people have stiff hips because they've never really worked the deep core muscles—abdominal, pelvic, and groin—that move their hips independent of their legs. Lovemaking is impeded when we cannot access and move these muscles because it is harder to perform the micromovements needed to rhythmically and repetitively press or massage a woman's inner and outer pleasure points. For a man, working these deep core muscles will enable him to better drop his hips (a movement referred to in this book as the Hip Drop) in a targeted forward and backward rocking motion rather than the straight pumping movements popularized in porn. For a woman, better hip articulation allows for better pelvic positioning, which helps her guide her lover to increase her (and his) pleasure.

In Eastern philosophy, it is understood that all movement emanates from the lower abdominal area called the hara. This life force is called Kundalini (sex) energy, and originates at the base of the spine in the first chakra. It then moves up the spine to the hara, the second chakra (also referred to as the sex or creative chakra), located just below the belly button. When not expressed somehow—either creatively, through love of family and friends, erotically, or through a passion that rewards you and opens your heart—this energy can become stagnant. The most powerful release of this sex energy is the orgasm. I have noticed from years of teaching that stiff hips are especially exemplified by people who find it difficult to dance or to express themselves in a sexual

Orgasm causes a release from the hip area up into the system, which relieves anxiety and tension as well as releasing Human Growth Hormone and testosterone into our system.

—DR. MEHMET OZ

or animal way. In fact, psychologist and biochemist Wilhelm Reich, who worked with Sigmund Freud and Carl Jung, confirmed what the ancient Tantrics had been saying for years about Kundalini energy: They believed that the inability to move this sexual energy because of social, cultural, and psychological constraints was the cause of most neurosis.

There are many social and psychological inhibitions associated with using our hips suggestively. Remember the controversy when "Elvis the Pelvis" hit the scene? CBS censors went so far as to insist that he be televised only from the waist up on *The Ed Sullivan Show*. Elvis's hip movements onstage drove the women in his audience (and probably a few guys) into a frenzy. Our society discourages us from learning to move our hips suggestively, and this often causes us to feel embarrassed or shameful about our sexuality. The inability to move our hips physically can also be a manifestation of our emotional and psychological state. Learning to loosen our hips will help loosen our hearts and minds—they are all connected! Remember, hearts, minds, and hips are all like parachutes: They work best when they're open.

In this chapter we will talk about how the hips move in relation to the spine, why this is important in increasing our sexual fluency, and give you some Love Locks to start warming up!

> "Culture is the enemy of Biology."
>
> —JOSEPH CHILTON PEARCE, AUTHOR OF *THE BIOLOGY OF TRANSCENDENCE*

THREE PLANES TO PARADISE

Allow me to introduce you to your hips (fig. 1). I like to think of the way we can learn to move our hips as having three very private planes to paradise: the **vertical**, the **lateral**, and the **horizontal**. Learning to move in these three planes, first alone and then in combination, will give you access to worlds you

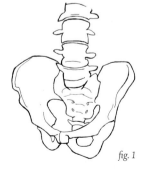

fig. 1

never thought possible. You will truly have two tickets to paradise that you can cash in anytime, and I can guarantee you'll soon be racking up those frequent-flyer miles. So strap yourself in.

VERTICAL: This up-and-down motion happens when your sacrum—the large triangular bone at the upper back wall of your pelvic cavity—rocks forward and backward from the lumbar spine. The Hip Drop movement (below) best exemplifies this.

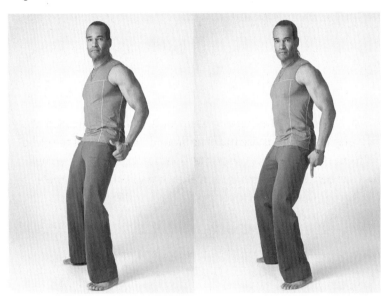

LATERAL: This motion is made when you lift your hips up toward your ribs and down, shifting the left or right iliac crest (the upper hip bone on your side) up and down using your oblique muscles (better known as your love handles). The Pendulum's windshield-wiper motion (opposite, top) demonstrates this well.

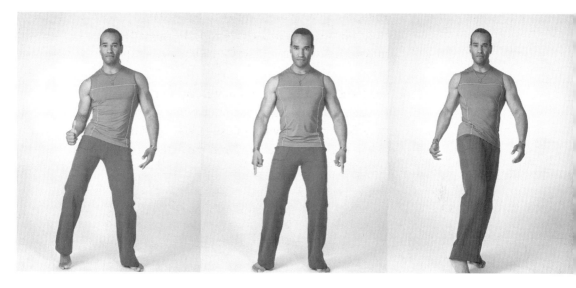

HORIZONTAL: The horizontal motion, sometimes called the transverse plane, is like traveling around the equator of the globe using the sacrum and coccyx (tailbone) at the base of the spine as your axis. The Revolver movement (below) is a great example.

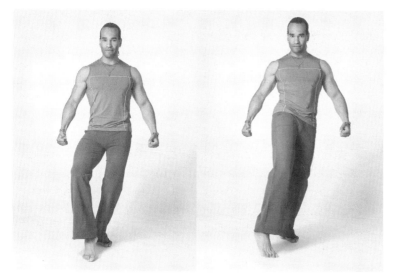

Of course, these movements can mix and mingle in myriad ways, but being able to refer to them as markers will be invaluable for you in moving with—and being moved by—your lover. For instance, the vertical forward and backward motion of the pubic bone, hinged at the lumbar, creates what we might call the motion of the ocean: a pelvic rocking motion essential for hitting the G-spot. A woman's vagina is actually tipped downward at a forty-five-degree angle when she is lying down, so the typical male ninety-degree, straight-in thrust literally misses everything of any real stimulation value for the woman. To stimulate the G-spot he actually needs an up-and-in motion. This is why it is helpful for the woman's hips to be lifted and her knees brought back; a pelvic tilt creates better access to the G-spot. If she holds and moves slightly in a pelvic tilt, and he does a pelvic rock with a dropping motion, the Fourth of July will arrive early and often. But more on all this later!

A full-body orgasm is like a full-on neuronal assault that moves through the heart like a sexy tsunami as it rushes up to the brain. The all-important pathway for this energy rush is your spine. This ascension of orgasmic energy ultimately heightens your sense of self and well-being.

THE LOVER'S SPINE: Love Locks

As important as it is to meet your hips, it is equally if not more important to meet your spine. The spine not only supports all of the muscles that we will be talking about but also plays a major role in our orgasmic abilities. Think of the spine as an energy highway that delivers orgasmic energy from the hara area to the brain. When the highway has roadblocks, there is a bottleneck of energy, and what could be a huge rush turns a love lock into a rush-hour gridlock. Stretching and strengthening the muscles that move and protect the lumbar vertebrae is of the utmost importance in improving sexual performance.

I like to think of the lumbar (the lower spine) as the love bar. This lower spine area includes all of the muscles between your diaphragm and your pelvis, including your lower abdominals, lower obliques, and transverse abdominus. (The glutes also play an important role in pelvic performance.) The lumbar portion of your spine bears the most body weight and also provides the most flexibility. All of the muscles surrounding and supporting the lower spine are the muscles that we use to move our hips.

Our mid-thoracic spine, including the serratus muscles that surround the ribs and the middle and upper abdominals (above the navel), are often employed as sexual default muscles because of lack of hip mobility. This mid-thoracic area and its muscles are actually designed more for rooting and stability: to help you hold positions during lovemaking so you can move your hips with more accuracy.

I developed spinal exercises that I call Love Locks out of my combined understandings of martial arts, dance, and Tantra. I originally learned elements of these positions during my martial arts training in China, where we practiced spinal locks to develop and sustain chi during kung fu, chi gong, and tai chi. I incorporated this

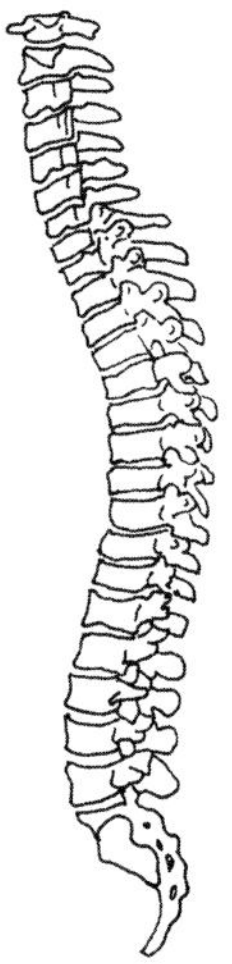

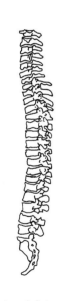

fig. 2

fig. 3

Lover's Spine

training into my dancing and learned to isolate the muscles that were needed to practice and perfect the moves. Later, when I was working with Tantra teachers in Maui, I realized that many of the martial arts movements were the same as the Tantric exercises I was learning (called *bandhas*). The Tantra teachers asked me how to train the muscles, not only to hold and perfect the *bandhas* but also to move their hips in a more effective way, and that was the beginning of the "Fit for Love" training program. By combining my experience and expertise in each area, I learned that the same muscles I had been training were invaluable in the intricate intimate isolations necessary to make love well. I discovered how micro movements could produce macro results.

Notice in the spine diagram how the lumbar vertebrae curve back (fig. 2). We want to train your lumbar to do the opposite—to curve up and under, creating a pelvic tilt. In order to get down and dirty, your hips have to move up and under, side to side, and around. Notice, too, how the thoracic spine (the area from the base of the neck to the top of the rib cage) has a natural slouch—ouch! In order to breathe better and create ample space for your lungs and heart, not to mention make your waistline smaller, you want your spine to curve the other way—to straighten and lift *up*, as shown in the Lover's Spine illustration (fig. 3). This position shows the spine holding a Love Lock position, which allows energy to flow more freely up and down your spine.

These lock positions can be practiced anywhere, anytime, without anyone else noticing. Many people who practice spine locks say they notice an immediate change in their energy level, and working with the energy flowing through your body is crucial to better sexual performance. Before sex, you can use the lock positions to develop energy. During sex, you can use them to sustain energy. Learn to breathe deeply during sex—especially when you feel an orgasm coming on—by circulating the energy down the front of your body on an inhale, and then up your spine and out on the exhale, and you're on the way to longer, stronger, and incredibly more satisfying sexual experiences. After sex, you can use spine locks to work with the energy you developed during sex. It's a little like sexual recycling!

Now let's look at the difference between the spine (fig. 2) and the Lover's Spine (fig. 3). Notice the difference between the normal female spine (fig. 4) and the posture-adjusted Female Lover's Spine (fig. 5), and the male spine (fig. 6) versus the Male Lover's Spine (fig. 7). Look at how the spine adjusts and straightens out to allow more energy to flow as the locking points are achieved.

You won't need a partner to practice these locks. Although they can be practiced individually, ultimately you want to be able to do them all at once (picture a flamenco dancer). Practicing them repeatedly will improve your posture, flatten your abs (especially your lower abs), and take inches off your waist. Remember, for women, hip-to-

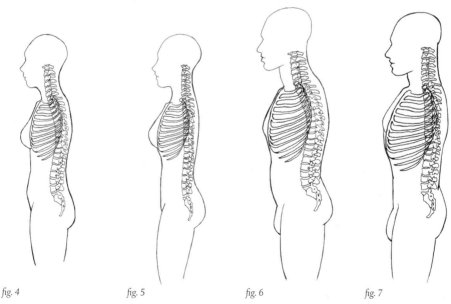

fig. 4   fig. 5   fig. 6   fig. 7

Female Lover's Spine   **Male Lover's Spine**

waist ratio depicts health and fertility, an evolutionarily sound attractor factor. For men, it is the shoulder-to-waist ratio.

What do we find attractive? Ultimately, in getting fit for love, one would seek an optimum evolutionary physical attractiveness ratio. Women tend to find men attractive who have a shoulder-to-waist ratio of 0.7, meaning that the man's waist is about 70 percent as wide as his shoulders. Men find women attractive who have a 0.7 hip-to-waist ratio, meaning that the woman's waist is about 70 percent as wide as her hips. This implies high fertility, which, even when people are not seeking to procreate, is a source of arousal and attractiveness in a lover. So practicing exercises that target the muscles in the waistline will not only make you better at sex, they will also make you sexier!

In some of these exercises, I will have you perform what may seem like an exaggerated pelvic tilt, but what you're doing is opening to full pelvic power. Achieving this full-tilt position is like opening the faucet to a full energy flow—and has the added advantage of bringing relief from most back pain, including sciatica. Being able to move into and hold a full tilt will enable you not only to work better with your own energy but also to open your lover to his or her energy. Remember, orgasms themselves are energy; they are seizures, energy overloads, sexy short circuits of our neural systems. If you want to intensify and lengthen these short circuits, you've got to lengthen and strengthen your spine. Check out what your spine looks like in the Full Tilt Spine position (fig. 8) compared to the normal spine (fig. 2, page 8).

Less pain and more pleasure? Sign me up for that program, right? Are you ready to go full tilt?

Check out the Female Lover's Full Tilt position and the Male Lover's Full Tilt (fig. 9). Notice how these full-tilt positions lift the sacrum and pubic bone up from their normal closed position to positions that are more open to giving and receiving pleasure. Under these circumstances, both the penis and the G-spot are easily accessible to meet and greet each other in amorous engagement. If you decide to take it deeper in a frontal entry position, the elevated pubic bones can more easily rub each other the right way.

Here are the locks and their benefits.

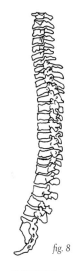

fig. 8

Full Tilt Spine

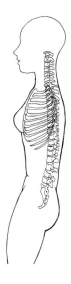

Female Lover's Full Tilt

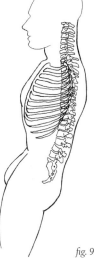

fig. 9

Male Lover's Full Tilt

SACRAL/COCCYX LOVE LOCK

ALSO KNOWN AS a Kegel exercise, this lock is accomplished by contracting the pubococcygeus (PC) muscles in your pelvic floor, the ones you use to "hold back" urination. By tightening up the PC muscles you pull on the coccyx (the tailbone at the base of the spine), hence the term pubococcygeus muscle. When you contract this muscle, you will feel a sweet sensation run up your spine to your head. This is called an orgasmic opening. When people have an orgasm, the PC muscle pulls and contracts, opening the gate through which the energy ascends upward and downward. The stronger this muscle, and the stronger the pull and pulse during orgasm, the stronger the orgasm. Practice contracting and holding these muscles six times a day for ten seconds. This extra minute will lead to hours of pleasure. Yup, better sex in sixty seconds.

LUMBAR LOVE LOCK

THIS IS DONE by contracting the lower abs and relaxing the lumbar spine. It's a great cure for lordosis (swayback) and, in many cases, sciatica. The Frog and Suitcase stretches (chapter 2) can help you prepare for this lock. Doing the various lower abdominal exercises will enhance your ability to do both the locks in this chapter and the all-important Hip Drops described in more detail in chapter 4.

1. Begin sitting or standing with your knees bent and your feet shoulders' width apart.
2. Inhale. As you exhale, contract your lower abdominal muscles, tucking your sacrum under and lifting your pubic bone up. As you do this, be aware of your lumbar spine opening as the vertebrae of the lower back open.

THORACIC LOVE LOCK

A GREAT CURE for bad posture, this lock is achieved by contracting the middle back and spine muscles to lift the ribs. Practicing the Abdominal (Ab) Stretch Heart Opener exercise (page 44) will help you perfect this lock.

1. Begin sitting or standing with your feet shoulders' width apart.
2. Engage the pelvic tilt (Lumbar Love Lock)
3. Inhale. As you exhale, using the mid-thoracic back and spine muscles, lift your ribs straight up away from your hips as if to lift your sternum (where your ribs connect in the center of your chest) away from your navel. Although it will move your shoulders back, *the movement is not done by moving your shoulder, but by lifting your heart.*

THE CERVIX LOVE LOCK

IN THIS LOCK you stretch the seventh vertebrae of the neck (beginning at the cervix) by drawing the top of your head up as you draw your chin directly back. The Cervix Love Lock is a great cure for kyphosis (hunchback). In detail:

1. Stand and place the backs of your shoulders against a wall.
2. Place the back of your head against the wall (use a folded towel behind your head if you wish).
3. Visualize drawing your chin straight back toward the wall as you lift the top of your head straight up toward the ceiling.

These Love Locks are an integral part of making love for both women and men, as they are also used to postpone orgasm and perpetuate the lovemaking process. As you feel an orgasm coming on, exaggerate the Sacral/Coccyx Love Lock and the Cervix Love Lock. The Thoracic Love Lock in the chest and Lumbar Lock are also employed, but do not need to be as pronounced. At this point it is also important to press your tongue to the roof of your mouth, as the whole process allows the energy of the orgasm to be brought up through your body. You can rapidly inhale and exhale or inhale, then exhale in short quick breaths. Try to feel the breaths deep in your lower abdomen. You can also let out a low, deep, drawn-out *ki* sound (pronounced "key"). All of these represent a kind of sexy CPR, a way to resuscitate yourself and bring new life to your lovemaking in the midst and throes of it.

Successful sex is about subtleties. It is about passionate, accurate articulations and expressions of the muscles surrounding the hips and lumbar spine, guided by aware, empathetic hearts and minds—only if you're interested in having and sharing earth-shattering orgasms, of course!

Take five—that is, take at least five minutes a day to practice all of the Love Locks at once. While you are holding the positions, place your tongue on the roof of your mouth and inhale through your nose and down the front of your body into your genitals. As you exhale, follow your breath up your spine, over your head, and out your mouth in a sort of relaxed sigh: aaaah! You can do this while sitting if you like; just remember to tuck the hips under, then lift and extend your spine up through your neck as if a string were pulling you up from the top of your head, pulling your jaw and chin in toward the back of your neck.

2

IT'S AN INSIDE JOB

*M*AKE NO MISTAKE about it, great sex is a religious experience. Think about it: What is the number-one thing people say in every language during orgasm? "Oh, God!" Orgasms release dopamine, serotonin, oxytocin, norepinephrine (epinephrine is the neurotransmitter released by meth), and other beneficial hormones that deliver a delicious chemical cocktail into your brain that can leave you in a drunken stupor. Dopamine is, after all, where the word "dope" comes from.

The key to phenomenal sex, in the physical sense, is to first learn how to access your lover's pleasure points—both the outer (such as the nape of the neck) and inner erogenous zones, sites in our bodies that are made up of nerve bundles. Next, learn how to repeatedly and rhythmically, passionately, and precisely stroke, press, and rub those areas. Both partners can contribute to this process by learning what movements work best for them and communicating these to their partner. Great sex requires syncing together into a relaxed rhythm. It's finding a fluid glide and slide, with smooth strokes that slip you both into a tantalizing trance. Great lovers find and fixate on these isolated inner nerve bundles; they pay attention to the nuances of their partner's breathing, how they are adjusting their body, and whether they are comfortable and relaxed. They are completely present with each other as they perpetuate their partner's arousal process. For the man, is she opening to and really receiving you? Is she comfortable and relaxed? Any and all positions are worthless if she is not comfortable, relaxed, and able to be fully present and feel your presence. In sex, more so than at any other time, body language is a barometer. Truly phenomenal sex is about intimacy, intricacy, and innocence that can take you into a silent wildness that shakes your souls beyond anything *Playboy* ever imagined.

So how do we achieve these orgasms? First, let's take a look at men's and women's sexual circuitry and erogenous zones. The inner erogenous zones are places where nerve endings bundle. It is very, very important to remember that nerve endings grow where attention and energy go. If you have difficulty locating a spot, remember the old adage: If at first you don't succeed, rub, rub again—and again! Erotic nerves are like Tantric tendrils reaching for the light. Once they find a source of nourishment, energy, and affection they seem to grow and reach toward it.

Dr. Jenny Wade said, "Basically the physical act of sex is simply the stimulation of nerve ends located at various erogenous structures." She argued that most women have "boregasms." I hope you will use the training and information in this book to change any boregasms or "snoregasms" into "moregasms"!

SEXUAL CIRCUITRY

Both men and women have a "fight or flight" (sympathetic) and a "rest and digest" (parasympathetic) nervous system. The spine houses the sympathetic pudendal, pelvic, and hypogastric nerves. The parasympathetic vagus nerve wanders outside the spine, ultimately connecting to the cervix and uterus in women, but is not connected directly to any sex organs in men. These nerves that run up, down, and around the spine are responsible for the creation and acknowledgment of our orgasms, so it is imperative that we obtain, protect, and maintain a healthy spinal and nervous system. Unnecessary and excess physical and emotional stress are not only bad for our immune system but also extremely detrimental to our sexual system. This is why practicing Love Locks is so important to our energy circulation and overall health.

The sexual hot spots we will be referring to are nothing more than areas in the human body where bundles of nerves hook up with sex organs. When these nerve bundles are stimulated through sexual activity, orgasm can result. Becoming familiar with your individual erotic wiring will help you and your partner better understand your bodies and how to turn each other on. By practicing and learning how to stimulate each of these areas, you can orchestrate some orgasmic masterpieces! All of these nerves are in some way interconnected, so by working with one, you are influencing them all. Pay attention and take your time with one another.

PUNDENDAL NERVE The woman's clitoris (fig. 10) and the male scrotum (fig. 11) are connected to the pudendal nerve. The pudendal nerve made the news some time ago when cyclists and spinners became impotent due to this nerve being compressed by their bike seat as they rode. The pudendal nerve runs through the perineum floor to the clitoris in women, and to the glans penis and penile skin and scrotum in men. It also stimulates the skin of the pelvic floor and anus; this is why the perineum massage is such a great appetizer and foreplay before the erotic entrée. Both the pudendal and the pelvic nerve enter the spinal cord at the upper sacrum, S2 to S4.

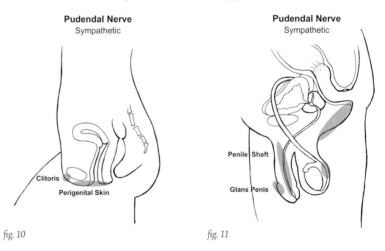

fig. 10   fig. 11

THE PELVIC NERVE The pelvic nerve is connected to the woman's vagina, including the G-spot, cervix, perineal floor, genital skin, and anus (fig. 12). In men it stimulates the head of the penis and the frenulum on the underside of the penis, the male version of the clitoris (fig. 13).

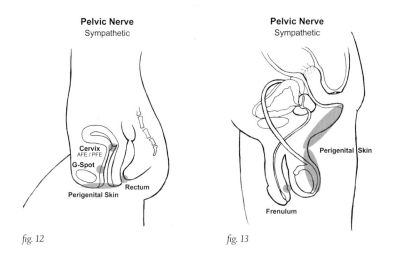

Pelvic Nerve
Sympathetic

Cervix
AFE / PFE
G-Spot
Perigenital Skin
Rectum

fig. 12

Pelvic Nerve
Sympathetic

Perigenital Skin
Frenulum

fig. 13

The hypogastric nerve stimulates the cervix and uterus in women (fig. 14) and the prostate and testes in men (fig. 15). It enters the spine between T10 and T12, just above the lumbar but close enough to influence it—an area known as the Thoracolumbar Erection Center. The hypogastric nerve enters the pelvic region at the back of the navel center, which is a main pivot point of the pelvis during sex.

THE HYPOGASTRIC NERVE

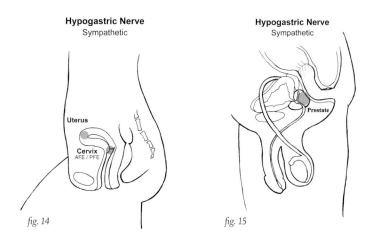

Hypogastric Nerve
Sympathetic

Uterus
Cervix
AFE / PFE

fig. 14

Hypogastric Nerve
Sympathetic

Prostate

fig. 15

THE VAGUS NERVE

For both men and women, the parasympathetic vagus nerve is responsible for our ability to relax. The nerve meanders throughout our system from the brain down the front of the body, working our organs such as our hearts, lungs, and digestive organs. We can all affect this nerve through meditation, contemplation, and basic relaxation and breathing techniques, which can help stabilize our system. Women, however, hit the nervous system jackpot because for them, the vagus nerve also runs through the uterus and cervix (fig. 16). In combination with the three other nerves we've discussed that make contact with the woman's sex organs, the vagus nerve allows her to have absolutely monstrous orgasms!

Vagus Nerve
Parasympathetic

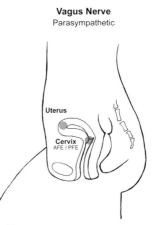

fig. 16

THE FEMALE CLITORIS is the only organ made specifically for sex. It houses eight to ten times the nerve endings of the male penis, although the frenulum works pretty well for us. It is a big mistake to ignore these areas in our efforts to arouse and satisfy our lovers.

FEMALE HOT SPOTS

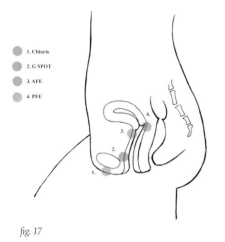

1. Clitoris
2. G SPOT
3. AFE
4. PFE

fig. 17

The **clitoris** is the most obvious and well-known area for achieving female climax. In my experience, it is not only an independent point of pleasure, as popularized, but also a conduit through which deeper, more powerful orgasms can be achieved. It can become an energy junction that ignites, amplifies, and significantly intensifies the potential of the inner pleasure points, leading to much more powerful "blended" orgasms.

The **G-spot** is a nerve plexus located about an inch or two into the vagina on the navel side, up and in behind the pubic bone. The texture of the skin at the G-spot is similar to that on the roof of the back of your mouth. It is the contact point of the pelvic nerve. This is a bit more potent in output than the pudendal nerve, which stimulates the clitoris, and so is capable of a more powerful orgasm. The G-spot, like a magic genie, may need to be rubbed into existence.

The **AFE**, or Anterior Fornix Erogenous zone, is the area at the top rear (navel side) of the vaginal canal in front of the cervix. (Although not shown here, note that the topmost rear crease of the cervix is called the Deep Spot or T-Zone, and is another potent stimulation point.)

The **PFE,** or Posterior Fornix Erogenous zone, is the area at the bottom rear of the vaginal canal in front of the cervix. (Note that the bottommost rear crease of the cervix is called the Cul de Sac, and is also a potent stimulation point.)

Warning: Any and all of these areas can shift slightly up, down, or to the left or right in the general vicinity where they were previously found. As the comedian Carlos Mencia said, "Honey, it's not my fault; it moved. It was there yesterday!"

> DEPENDING ON THE woman, the G-spot may be a bit to the left or right side. A woman can use the horizontal plane motion of her hips to present her man with an angle that works for her.

MALE HOT SPOTS

EXTERNAL

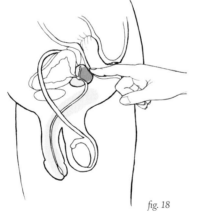

fig. 18

The **frenulum** is the arrowhead point at the underside of the penis head. It is similar to the female clitoris, but with fewer nerve endings, and is innervated by the pelvic nerve. It is a very sensitive area, so ladies, be generous with the tongue and please be gentle with the teeth.

INTERNAL

The **prostate**, or P-spot, is straight ahead through the anus about two inches in (as seen in diagram). Like a woman's G-spot, it can be responsible for incredibly powerful orgasms. Considering it holds thirty percent or more of a man's semen, ejaculations are increased markedly when the prostate is included in the stimulation process. The prostate can be externally stimulated in the area of the diagram where the middle finger's knuckle is located, in what is sometimes called the "million-dollar spot." It is innervated by the hypogastric nerve, which enters at the Thoracolumbar Erection Center, T10 through L2. It is operated by the same nerve center that allows the prostate to close off urine while the penis is erect and semen about to be ejaculated.

Your P-spot is your He-spot, so take care of your prostate. Saw palmetto, pygeum, and pumpkinseed oil seem to work well for me—these usually come in pill or gel form, and if taken daily they stabilize the cell structure and protect the prostate from enlarging. It has also been suggested that they improve sexual performance; I have noticed an enjoyable difference. Check with your doctor or pharmacist before using these supplements, and get regular prostate exams if you are over forty years old.

STAGES OF AROUSAL

It has long been thought that there were four stages in sexual activity. Now it is understood that these four must be preceded by a fifth: desire, which is created by both internal and external stimulation. Internally, your level of testosterone is directly related to your desire, or libido. Dopamine levels or the thought of possible pleasure also increases desire. External stimulation is that which you desire—your lover. After desire, the four stages are:

Arousal, when the woman begins to "get wet" and the man erect. Lips and nipples swell as the partners prepare for a sexual encounter.

Plateau, just before orgasm (if there is one). When people get aroused to this point, they should perpetuate this stage as long as possible to build the potency of the orgasm. Plateau is a stage of constant arousal and rearousal.

Orgasm, when a person is brought over the edge into climactic convulsions and release.

Refractory period, when the partners return to prearousal form.

ORGASMS

Most twentieth-century sex experts, from Alfred Kinsey to Masters and Johnson, agreed that there were four types of female orgasms: clitoral, vaginal, blended, and multiple orgasms. Since those early years of sexual studies, understandings of the female orgasm have been expanded. With the introduction of Tantra to the West and information from modern sex experts such as Dr. Jenny Wade (author of *Transcendent Sex*) and Dr. Ruth Westheimer, we can now add to the list the cervical orgasm, the extended orgasm (a prolongation of any of the aforementioned), and the much-debated female ejaculation.

The purpose of *Fit for Love* is to help you combine my insights with your newly acquired physical skills and abilities so you can achieve orgasms beyond anything ever imagined or achieved by our prophetic predecessors. I myself have explored and experimented with wonderful success, so I know from experience that you, too, can extend a blended orgasm. You, too, can extend multiple orgasms and top them off with a female ejaculation. You, too, can reach new places within and with your lover, and you may discover things on your own that I have not. Please share as I have!

Here is a brief description of each type of female orgasm.

Clitoral orgasm, when a woman "comes," occurs when the clitoris is stimulated. Clitoral orgasms are also called peak orgasms because they usually reach a peak and then decline. This kind of orgasm is attached to the pudendal nerve (fig. 10, page 20) and is usually localized to the pelvic area.

A **vaginal** orgasm is one that involves the G-spot. Although not as powerful as a cervical orgasm, it is strong enough to cause deep quaking and tremors. The G-spot is stimulated by the pelvic nerve (fig. 12, page 21).

A **cervical** orgasm involves the AFE, located just above the cervix, or the PFE, located just below the cervix. It is sometimes referred to as a valley orgasm because it is like a deep, moving riptide that pulls a woman in and under, where she implodes into herself. The cervix has three main nerves: the pelvic (fig. 12, page 21), the hypogastric (fig. 14, page 21), and the powerful vagus nerve (fig. 16, page 22). The uterus also has the hypogastric nerve. Remember, the orgasm is a pleasuring power surge through these nerves, up your spine to your brain. In talking about the AFE and PFE it is important to note that, because they are located at the cervix, any one, if not all three, of these nerves can contribute to an erotic eruption from these erogenous zones. These nerves can also branch off to form new points of pleasure as they awaken.

The **blended** orgasm is a combination of two orgasms involving the clitoris and an internal stimulation point. I like to call it an AC/DC: The internal orgasm is like an oscillating alternating current that permeates body and being, while the clitoral orgasm is more like a direct current.

UNLESS SHE GETS chafed or becomes overly sensitive, a woman is often just warming up once she's had her first orgasm. This is why the man should postpone his ejaculation and prolong his refractory period as long as possible—if he decides to release at all.

A **multiple** orgasm can be a sequence of one orgasm after another, or one within another. It can be a few in a row, or a small one leading to a larger one. It can be a large earthquake followed by tremors. Again, a woman's partner must pay attention to where she is during the orgasm and where stimulation is most needed to perpetuate the orgasms once they begin.

The **extended blended** is an "übergasm" that during its fade-out is restimulated into another one using a different internal stimulation point (with or without the clitoris). Every woman is different, but in my experience, any orgasm can serve as an ignition point for others.

The **multiple extended blended,** which for lack of a better name I call the "superübergasm," can occur after an extended blended orgasm by reinitiating stimulation almost immediately afterward, using butterfly kissing on a sensitive clitoris to help reignite an internal point. Here, again, if the woman is open to multiple restimulations her partner can alternate between internal and external stimulation points. This can seem like a never-ending, escalating experience that goes on and on until every cell and fiber of the woman's being is engaged and engorged. She will feel wonderfully ravished and wrecked afterward, but her smiles and giggles will say it all.

Female ejaculation, or "fejaculation," is usually the result of G-spot stimulation, although some women can achieve it through clitoral stimulation. Some studies have found nerves connecting the clitoris and the G-spot. The debate mentioned earlier is not whether or not women are capable of emitting an ejaculate, but what the nature of the fluid is: urine or not urine? According to Mary Roach, in her bestseller *Bonk: The Curious Coupling of Science and Sex*, "It's possible some women expel urine, others a prostatic fluid, and some a mixture. The debate drags on."

In *The Science of Orgasm*, the scholars Barry Komisaruk, Carlos Beyer-Flores, and Beverly Whipple explain that, from the time of Hippocrates, doctors have stimulated women with a medical (or pelvic) massage to treat so-called hysteria. The medical massage was meant to induce a "hysterical paroxysm" otherwise known as an orgasm. According to historian Rachel Maines in *The Technology of Orgasm*, treating hysteria with medical massage was "the job no one wanted." How times have changed!

A **female ejaculation plus,** or **fejac plus,** involves multiple orgasms accompanied by an ejaculation. This can include both clitoral and vaginal orgasms and can last a long, long time. As this is a deliberate occurrence, be sure, if you plan on summoning one, to keep extra towels handy. Yes, I said "summoning," because this is an otherworldly experience.

Note that when a woman has an extended blended, multiple extended blended, or fejac plus orgasm she may have a difficult time communicating, as her brain has literally gone into sensory overload through seizure. Give her some time to reenter the atmosphere. Chilling her with light, ticklelike touches all over her body, soft kisses, even light pulls on her hair and light nibbles is often greatly appreciated, as she is hypersensitive. Every nerve ending and pore is open and aroused.

Now, here's the story on male orgasms:

Ejaculation is the release of semen, also known as "coming." It is usually stimulated by arousing the frenulum (the pelvic nerve—fig. 13, page 21) or the shaft (the pudendal nerve—fig. 11, page 20).

The **frenulum** orgasm, like the clitoral orgasm for women, is what I personally consider "coming." It is usually accompanied by ejaculation, and although it's enjoyable, we should in no way think this is it! In Tantric practice men are taught, through breathing and spinal elongation (Love Locks) to postpone ejaculation in order to increase the intensity of the experience.

The **P-spot** or **He-spot** orgasm is a drawing up from inside that will ride up a man's spine and explode in his brain (this is what is meant by "mind-blowing"). It will literally rattle his teeth: It will seem like it's never going to stop coming, and he won't want to. A massage of the prostate internally or externally through the perineum adds greatly to this experience. The prostate can be stimulated externally in that million-dollar indentation just in front of the anus, if a man is not comfortable with a woman going "procto" on him. Since the prostate is stimulated by the hypogastric nerve (fig. 15, page 21), and the frenulum is stimulated by the pelvic nerve, the two together form a blended orgasm for men.

Every man should spend time talking with a lesbian about how to please a woman, and every woman should spend time talking with a gay man on how to please a man. These are women and men who share the intense experience of dealing with an erotic apparatus similar to their own. Lesbian women know more about the vagina, at least sexually, than most OB-GYNs, and gay men know more about the prostate sexually than most proctologists—what a wonderful resource.

GETTING STARTED:
Warm-up Stretches

Do you know what the number-one sex organ is? That's right—it's your brain. Your orgasm begins and ends in the brain by sending signals up your spine. So if you have a misaligned spine, the orgasm signals can be impeded or weakened, and if the muscles in your hips, glutes, and spine are tight, they are holding onto energy that could be used to power, intensify, and increase your orgasmic potential. With these simple stretches, you can not only alleviate physical discomfort and pain, but also create the opportunity for significantly more pleasure. Just as it is important to open the heart and free the mind in order to achieve great sex, it is also important to prepare the muscles, nerves, and neural pathways through which the orgasmic energy will travel. You want to enlist every available nerve to send those orgasmic surges of energy to explode in the brain! Remember, too, that contracting muscles in the perineum (pelvic floor) pump energy up the spine to the brain, so the better the condition of these muscles, the more intense the orgasm.

Warming up these muscles is important. In the gym, the first couple sets of reps for a muscle are preparation for the last set. In the final set you want to burn that muscle into oblivion so that when you finally stop and let go, you move from agony into ecstasy . . . sound familiar? This is why, when people move from machine to machine and never feel the burn, they don't get results. Being able to withhold an orgasm and withstand pain are two sides of the same coin. If you cannot sustain through the pain in the weight room, you won't be able to delay gratification and gain new pleasure in the bedroom.

Please don't take this to mean that you need to hurt yourself to get results! Try each of the stretches and exercises below and decide what works best for you. It is not necessary to do them all; you can pick and choose, mix and match, like the food groups. Try to practice at least one vertical, horizontal, and lateral stretch every day to increase your potency and energy flow. Then, to build up your strength, practice one exercise and/or dance movement from each group every other day. Some of these exercises may become strenuous at times, so please check with a physician if you have any concerns about your health before trying any and all exercises. I recommend performing these exercises on a yoga or Pilates mat. You can try doubling the mat for any exercises that you feel need a little more support under your back, butt, or knees.

Use this training as a way to come into understanding of yourself, a meditation to get inside your body. We know more about our cell phones, microwaves, and cars than we know about the one piece of equipment we can't trade up or trade in—our body. While you exercise, notice what sensations are occurring in your body. Remember what you're working toward: the ability to achieve new levels of sexual satisfaction. As the saying goes, failing to prepare is preparing to fail. You are preparing, practicing, and priming yourself for pleasure.

Try these exercises and dance movements to your favorite music. Believe me, you want to learn to move to rhythm, because establishing an intimate rhythm with your lover is key to bypassing the "fight or flight" response that halts any possibility of orgasm. Establishing a rhythm also keeps you within the proper proximity of the pleasure points. The beat, the rhythm is not just to keep time; it is also to keep space. If you move at a certain tempo, you can only cover so much space, area, or distance. Considering the size of the erogenous zones within a woman (about the size of a dime or quarter), it is important not to lose contact by moving too far one way or another. By the time you establish a rhythmic beat with your lover, you should have established a rhythmic space as well. A good example of this is scratching a mosquito bite: The area of a bug bite is only so big, so the slower the scratch tempo, the more accurate the scratch and the faster the relief. In our case the more accurate the rub, the faster the release (for the woman, of course). This understanding will become clearer in the "Turn on a Dime" section in chapter 5 (page 192).

Music is a great opportunity to practice tandem motions like the Milkshake and the Double Deep Drag, first by yourself and then with your lover. All rely on rhythm, precision, and passionate perseverance until the point of pleasure, the orgasmic escalation, presents itself.

It is also important to remember to be present for yourself and your lover, especially you guys! Often, in our society, the word *sensitive* can mean wimpy to some people. Here, you are not so much called upon to be sensitive as to be present and aware. When you are both present and accounted for in your own body, you will be in a much better position to feel and move in tandem with your partner's body.

Both in practicing these exercises and in intimate encounters with your lover, *feel* each movement. Don't just robotically go through the motions; take your time and enjoy the journey. You are alive! Learn to take pleasure in the process. Only then will you notice the nuances and subtleties that will lead to a sublime experience.

I will talk about a pelvic tilt often throughout this book, because it is an essential part of being fit for love. In the photo on the left I demonstrate a neutral pelvic tilt. Notice my hips are tucked under and up. In the photo on the right I show an increased pelvic tilt. Whenever engaging in a pelvic tilt, try to keep your navel close to your spine.

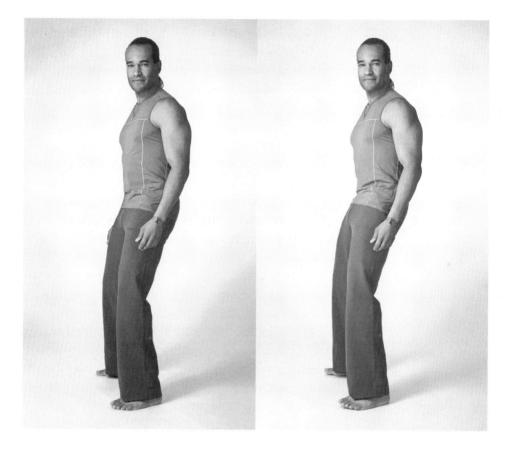

BACK STRENGTHENER, STANDING OR SEATED

THIS EXERCISE WILL strengthen your back and help eliminate lower-back soreness and fatigue. It also opens up your Thoracic Love Lock, improves your posture and breathing capacity, and provides a noticeable slimming of the waist.

1. Begin seated or standing with your knees outside your shoulders, supporting yourself with your hands in a pelvic tilt.

2. Inhale. As you exhale, arch your back up slightly and try to first extend one arm, then lower your arch. As you arch your back slightly up again, try to extend the other arm, still supporting yourself with the other arm. Notice the arching movement comes from the middle back and spine as opposed to the lumbar area, which is kept still and supported at all times. For beginners, always use your hands to support your body weight throughout these exercises until you feel strong enough to extend both hands at once either to the front or the side. You may even want to start by walking your hands up and down your legs, holding your shins.

3. As you feel stronger, inhale and try to touch the floor.

4. Then exhale and slowly try lifting your ribs slightly and your arms straight out to the side.

5. As you progress and feel stronger, try to extend your arms slowly out to the front again.

NOTE: *Try alternating your arms from the front or to the side as a variation. You will notice fatigue in the middle of your back. If you feel pain in the lower back, stop or try the movement with your hands on your knees again.*

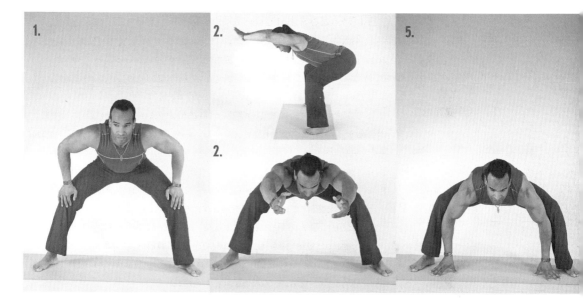

1.
2.
5.
2.

IN THE BEDROOM, a man needs to warm a woman up, like an oven, before he even thinks about entering her. As Ian Kerner argues in *She Comes First: The Thinking Man's Guide to Pleasuring a Woman*, it's important for a woman to feel she is capable and ready to be brought to orgasm, and more important that the man cares enough to give her one. I think of this as a kind of sexual chivalry, ensuring that a good knight will have a great night!

FORWARD FROG LUMBAR STRETCH

BYE-BYE BACK PAIN, hello pleasure! This stretch is the holy grail of hip motion. It allows you to move up and into position like nothing before, while alleviating all kinds of lumbar tightness and pain. This opens up the Lumbar Love Lock and allows you to prepare for the important Hip Drop and Deep Press (pages 132 and 140).

1. Start by sitting on the floor, your back straight and erect.
2. Place your feet out in front of you, heels together.
3. Create a pelvic tilt, bringing your navel toward your spine.
4. Move your feet far enough out so that you can just barely reach your heels with your completely outstretched arms.
5. Relax and inhale. As you exhale, place your hands, palms up, underneath your ankles.
6. Inhale. As you exhale, doing almost a bicep curl with your arms, begin pulling yourself forward and down.
7. Keep your head up and lead with your heart. When you can't move forward any farther with your heart, guide your head down toward your feet to complete the stretch.
8. Slowly release the stretch and repeat steps 6 and 7 as needed.

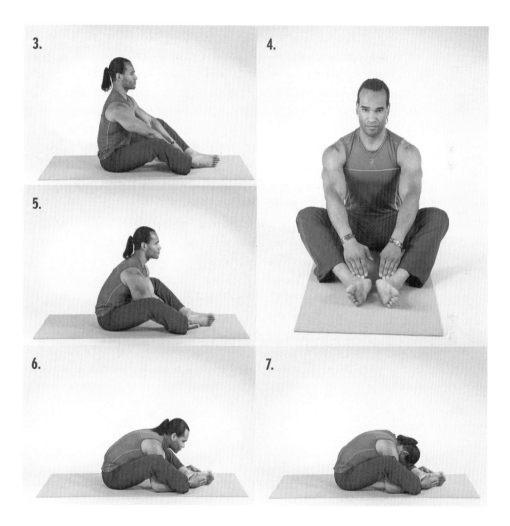

CHAIR FROG LUMBAR STRETCH

IF YOUR BACK is sore, injured, or just stiff, sit in a chair with your feet shoulders' width apart. Doing this stretch from a chair lets gravity do the work for you. Opening the Lumbar Love Lock is great for relieving back pain. The slow aided release of walking your hands down your shins is great in the office or on long plane rides.

1. Begin slowly inhaling and exhaling.
2. Create a pelvic tilt, bringing your navel toward your spine.
3. Place your hands on your knees.
4. Inhale. As you exhale, begin walking your hands down your shins, easing yourself slowly into the stretch about two inches at a time.
5. You should start to feel your lower-back muscles respond to the stretch and slowly loosen up as you go. You want to try to get your ribs and torso down to and eventually between your quads. If you can reach your feet, your back is in pretty good shape.
6. Release by slowly walking yourself back up. Slowly repeat steps 4 and 5 as needed.

If you feel any sharp pain during any of these exercises or stretches, stop immediately. If moved into too quickly, which we all do when we get excited over new possibilities, an exercise may be a little more than we can handle at the start. Be aware of any preexisting injuries when embarking on any new exercise, and take it slow. Nobody knows your body better than you, so it's up to you find your edge but not to jump over it!

STANDING HIP AND GLUTE STRETCH

OH, DOES THIS feel good—no more tight butt or stiff back! Creating more flexibility in your lower back and glutes loosens your hips, which in turn gives you more fluidity of movement in the bedroom.

1. Stand with feet a bit more than shoulders' width apart.
2. Engage a pelvic tilt.
3. Lift your left foot and place it across your right knee so that your left ankle is just above and outside your right kneecap.
4. Inhale. As you exhale, sink your right hip down toward your right heel.
5. Maintaining a pelvic tilt, lean forward and extend your arms. (Hold on to something for balance if you need to.) Hold for ten seconds.
6. Repeat with the other leg.

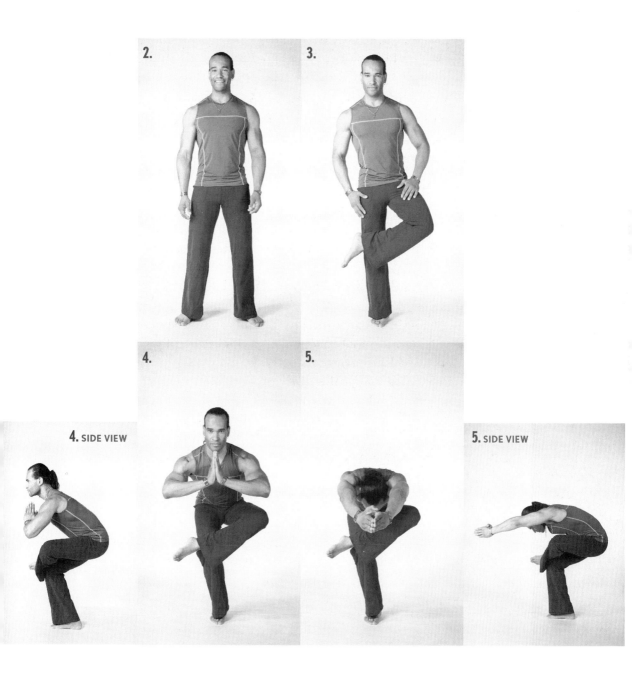

2.

3.

4.

5.

4. SIDE VIEW

5. SIDE VIEW

ABDOMINAL (AB)
STRETCH HEART OPENER

THIS STRETCH IS amazing for opening up the Thoracic Love Lock. Many people come to my class just to experience the release of the tension held in the emotional center, just beneath the sternum (breastbone). That is the heart chakra, after all! This stretch complements the Back Strengthener.

1. Sit with your knees bent and the small of your back pressed against the floor.
2. Take a ball (a child's kickball is good) and hold it just below your scapulae (shoulder blades) in the center of your back.
3. Gently lie down over the ball, with your arms down by your sides.
4. Try holding your arms out to the sides.
5. Try holding your arms over your head, clasping your elbows.
6. Try lifting your arms over the top of your head.
7. If working with a partner, have your partner press down on the left hip and the right shoulder as you exhale, causing a nice diagonal cross-body stretch. Lying on the ball releases the emotional tension held in the shoulder and sternum areas, so you can actually feel your heart release and open.

IN THE EAST, the development and perpetuation of an orgasm riding up the spine is believed to stimulate the chakras. The Western equivalent of each chakra is a gland, which releases a hormone that contributes to health, growth, and repair throughout the body.

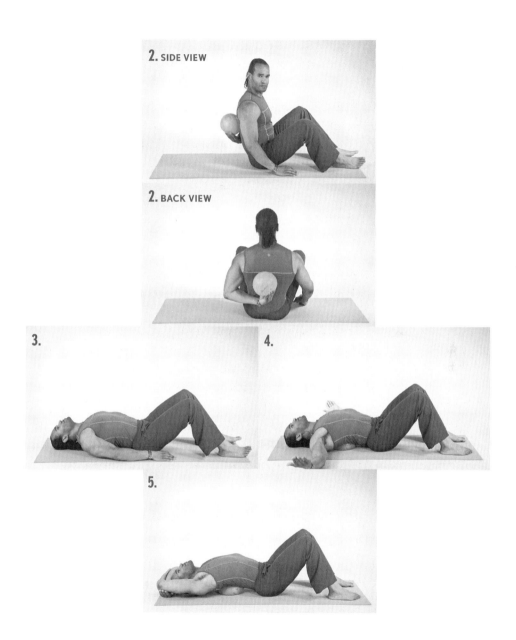

2. SIDE VIEW

2. BACK VIEW

3.

4.

5.

MODIFIED COBRA ABDOMINAL STRETCH

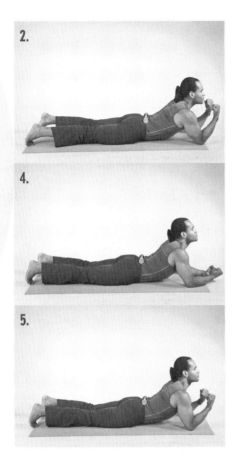

2.

4.

5.

THIS MODIFIED VERSION of the traditional yogic Snake Pose protects your lower back while stretching your abs. It is a great heart opener because it stretches deep into the abdominals and really enables and enhances the Thoracic Love Lock.

1. Lie facedown on the floor, stretched out with the soles of your feet facing up. Place your hands on the floor by your shoulders and hold your arms close to your sides as if preparing to do a push-up.

2. Press your waist and navel to the floor. *Do not let them come off the floor.* I sometimes place a weight on my lower back above my navel to keep me from lifting my waist.

3. Now, support yourself on your elbows, slightly in front of your body.

4. Inhale. As you exhale, pull your elbows down and back as if digging into the floor.

5. Slowly begin lifting your ribs forward and up from your sternum, leading with your heart. You should feel a stretch deep into your abdominals.

MODIFIED PIGEON WITH A TWIST

THIS EXERCISE IS a great release for tension in the hips, glutes, and lower back.

1. Lie facedown on the floor.
2. Pull your navel toward your spine and prop your torso up with your arms and hands as if beginning to do a push-up.
3. Bring your right knee forward, toward your chest, so that your right heel is beneath your right hip flexor. *Be sure your foot is not tucked inside your crotch.*
4. Lay your body down across your leg, with your left arm forward and out.
5. Extend your right arm out to the side. You should notice stretching in your right hip and glute.
6. Lift your right arm to your side and gently begin propping your body up on the right side (as if doing a one-arm push-up), increasing the stretch in your hip, back, and spine.
7. Repeat on the other side.

STANDING TRANSVERSE TWIST

THIS IS A modified Tai Chi/Chi Gong movement. In my class we use it as a great warm-up.

1. Begin with your feet a little more than shoulders' width apart.
2. Bend your knees and engage a pelvic tilt.
3. Hold your arms out to the sides, letting your shoulders drop down relaxed.
4. Straighten your spine by lifting your ribs up and away from your hips.
5. With your spine straight, try to swing your shoulder in front of your nose without moving your hips, first one way and then the other.
6. Continue until you feel your spine loosening.

FIND THE "FIT for Love" exercises that fit your and your lover's needs and practice, practice, practice!

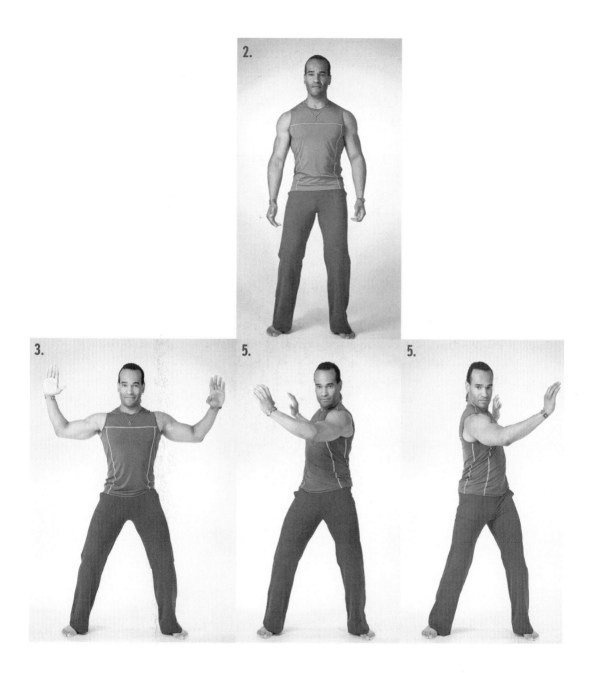

FACEDOWN TWIST OF FATE

THE FACEDOWN TWIST of Fate is a hip and back stretch that people just love, sometimes too much! During class I usually lose about fifty percent of my students to la-la land on this one. Perfect for beginners, it may be one of the most relaxing stretches ever.

1. Lie down on your side, relaxing on the elbow of the side you're lying on.
2. Lift your bottom leg up perpendicular to your body and lay it on the floor in front of you, bent at a ninety-degree angle.
3. Support yourself with your top arm. Stretch your bottom arm out in back of you. (You may want to put a folded towel or pillow beneath your head.)
4. Inhale. As you exhale, slowly lie down and reach your left arm out across in front of you.
5. Feel your back stretch, relax, and hold. Enjoy lying there for a while, then release.
6. To increase the stretch, try placing your top leg over your bottom leg.
7. Repeat on the other side.

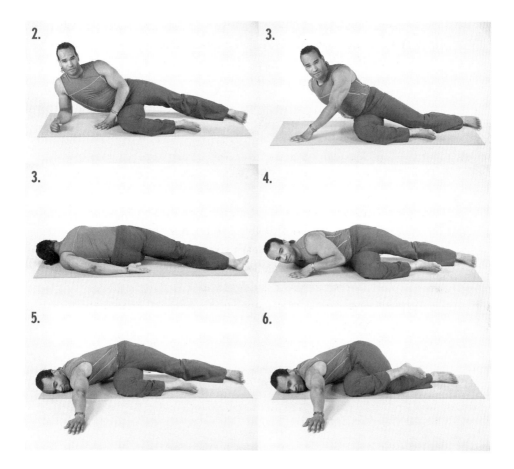

TWIST OF FATE

THE TWIST OF Fate is a soothing hip and back stretch that often gives you a chiropractic adjustment minus the chiropractor, because it allows multiple ways to adjust for different muscle stretches.

1. Lie on your back on the floor, shoulders flat.

2. Engage a pelvic tilt.

3. Keeping both shoulders flat on the floor and your right leg straight, lift your left knee up and over to the right (perpendicular to the body), bending your knee at a ninety-degree angle.

4. Use your right hand to try to guide your left knee down toward the floor. In the photo I am using a small weight to increase the stretch, but this is not necessary.

5. Repeat on the other side.

FROM NINON DE Lenclos, the famous French courtesan: "It takes more skill to make love than to maneuver an army!"

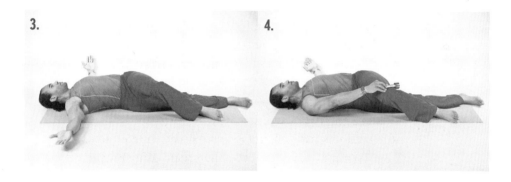

3.

4.

In physical therapy, weights are often used to stabilize or hold a joint in place while it heals. Here, we can use weights to help heal our occasional inflexibility. Try using them in different areas to enhance flexibility when you need a little more of a stretch than you're getting.

LEG-OVER TWIST OF FATE

THIS STRETCH ALLOWS you to go deep into the hip and glutes for a nice release.

1. Lie on your back on the floor, shoulders flat.
2. Engage a pelvic tilt.
3. Keeping both shoulders flat on the floor and your right leg straight, lift your left knee up, bending your leg at a ninety-degree angle and over to the right (over your right leg).
4. Pull your right leg up from under your left and place your right knee on top of your left knee, using your right hand to guide your right knee down. (In the final position you are lying on your right side with your right knee crossed over the top of your left knee.)
5. Repeat on the other side.

3.

4.

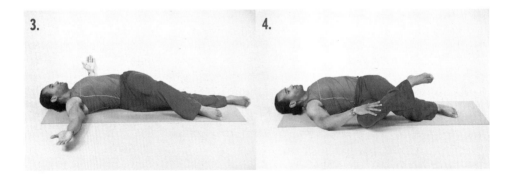

LEG-UNDER TWIST OF FATE

THIS STRETCH GETS into your sides and waistline.

1. Lie on your back on the floor, shoulders flat.

2. Engage a pelvic tilt.

3. Keeping both shoulders flat on the floor and your right leg straight, lift your left knee up and over to the right (perpendicular to the body), bending your knee at a ninety-degree angle.

4. With your left knee still over your right knee, use your right hand to try to guide your left knee down.

5. Repeat on the other side.

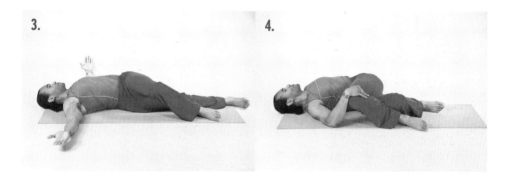

3.

4.

STANDING LATERAL STRETCH

THIS STRETCH FEELS great and will help improve your lateral lovin' motion.

1. Stand with your knees slightly bent, feet a little wider than shoulders' width apart.
2. Engage and *always* maintain a pelvic tilt.
3. Lift your arms above your head, holding your elbows with opposite hands.
4. Maintaining your pelvic tilt, inhale. As you exhale, lean to one side as far as you can. Lift your other rib toward the ceiling, away from your hip.
5. Maintaining your pelvic tilt, lean your torso toward the center, as if trying to bring your sternum down toward your navel.
6. Maintaining your pelvic tilt, inhale. As you exhale, lean to the other side as far as you can. Lift your other rib toward the ceiling, away from your hip.
7. Without coming straight back up, repeat steps 4, 5, and 6.

This stretch is also great to practice against a wall: Lean against a wall with your knees bent, the small of your back against the wall. Repeat steps 3 through 7.

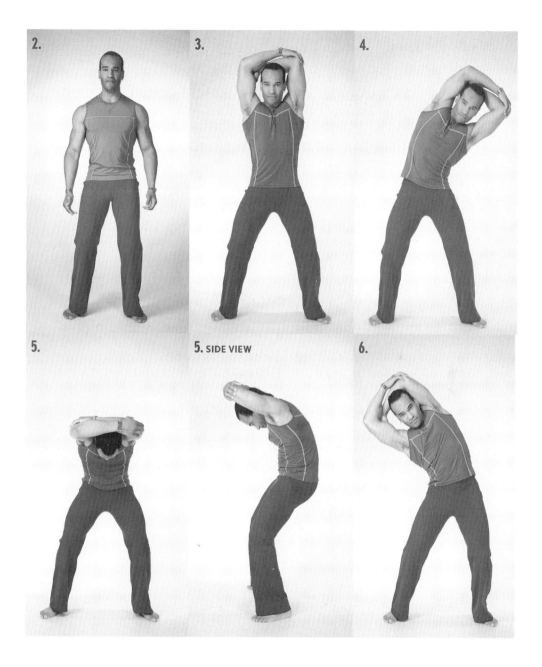

HIP FLEXOR (PSOAS STRETCH)

OH, DOES THIS stretch open you up. It really helps people whose hips are tight from sitting at a desk all day, and it can help relieve lower-back pain caused by a tight psoas (the muscle connecting your hip to your spine) pulling on the spine.

1. Kneel on your right knee with your left knee up, creating a box with your legs.
2. Turn your back (right) calf to the left so it makes a perpendicular angle with the front, creating an L shape. Place your left forearm on your left leg. Try to square your hips and keep them facing forward toward the left knee throughout. It should feel as if you are constantly trying to pull your left foot and heel forward. You want to lean your left knee forward, straight ahead, while keeping the right leg rooted and still.
3. Engage a pelvic tilt and reach your right arm over your head.
4. Sliding the front (left) foot forward a little, inhale. As you exhale, use your left heel, leading with your left knee, to pull your hips forward without moving your back (right) knee.
5. As you do this, keeping the pelvic tilt engaged, try to gently lean to your left, little by little. Your right leg will angle forward as your hip moves forward.
6. Repeat on the opposite side.

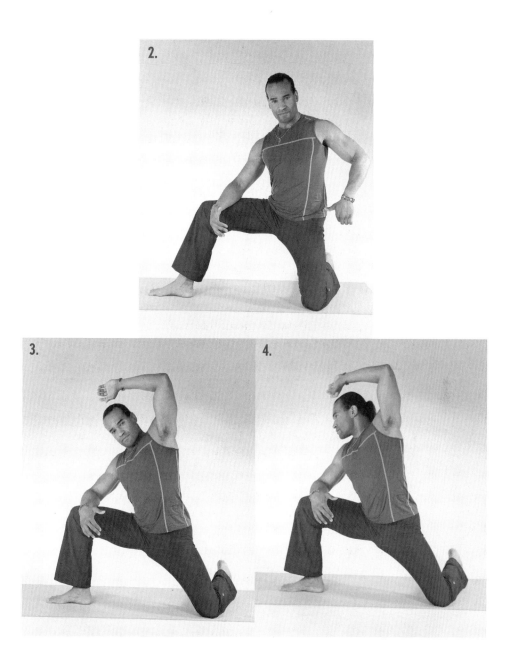

QUADRATUS LUMBORUM AND SPINALIS STRETCH (Q STRETCH)

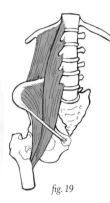

fig. 19

THIS IS A sweet stretch that opens up the back and spine, especially the often difficult quadratus muscle. You and your lover are going to love the lateral motions this stretch will allow you to make. Notice in the illustration (fig. 19) how the quadratus attaches the last rib to the hip. Because it can either help or hinder back strength, flexibility, and mobility, it is especially important to take care of it.

1. Sit on the floor, your back straight and erect.
2. Place your feet out in front of you, heels together.
3. Create a pelvic tilt, bringing your navel toward your spine.
4. Move your feet far enough out so that you can just barely reach your heels with your completely outstretched arms.
5. Inhale. As you exhale, begin leaning to your left.
6. Reach your right hand under your right leg from the inside out.
7. Inhale. As you exhale, try to reach your left hand across in front of you to hold your right hand.
8. Inhale. As you exhale, reach your left hand and arm in back of your head, trying to hold your right hand.
9. As you feel your hip and back stretch, try to keep your right shoulder down on the floor. Gently move into, but do not force, the stretch. Try to keep your hips, head, right leg, and foot in a straight line.
10. Repeat on the other side.

BEING TIGHT, STIFF, and experiencing limited mobility and inhibited range of motion are a just a few things many people in my gym talk about. Others complain about lack of strength and coordination. These movements will help you loosen up, tone up, and move in areas and ways you never knew you could—or needed to.

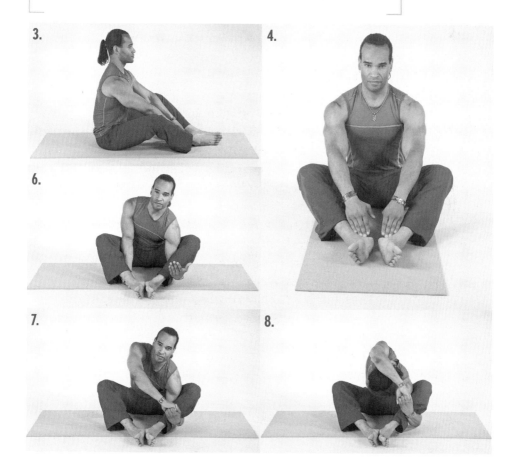

3.

4.

6.

7.

8.

NECK AND SHOULDER STRETCH

EVERYBODY LOVES THIS stretch because it gets rid of neck and shoulder tension and stress-induced pain almost immediately. Start with the most painful side first! If the pain is in your left rear neck or shoulder, you need to move your head in the opposite direction, to the right front. By loosening up the muscles around the neck and shoulders, you are helping to prepare for your Cervical Spine Love Lock, which can also help you decrease the effects of kyphosis. (Kyphosis, or forward head syndrome or hunchback, is common among those of us hunched over our computers all day.)

1. Stand, kneel, or sit relaxed.
2. With your right hand, reach around the back of your head and place your right hand on the left rear corner of your head.
3. Drop your shoulders down, especially your left shoulder. If you can, it will be beneficial to hold a weight or the side of a chair with your left hand.
4. Inhale. As you exhale, begin gently pulling your head with your right hand forward and down to the right, as if trying to bring your right ear to your right armpit.
5. If you are stretching with a partner, he or she can help you gently pull your head forward and down, applying minor pressure on your left shoulder. Your partner can even massage your left neck and shoulder area while guiding your head down.

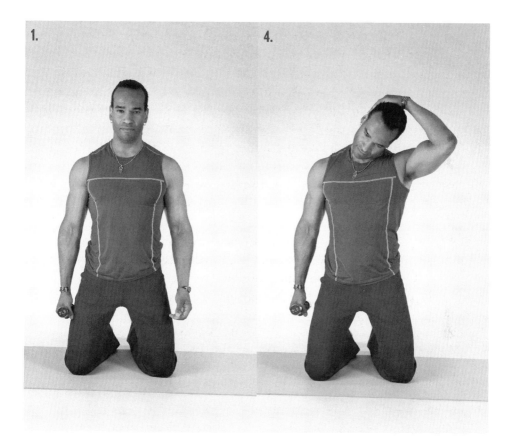

PELVIC PERINEUM STRETCH (HIP OPENER)

YOU MIGHT NOTICE a warm sensation moving through your body in this position. The Pelvic Perineum Stretch is a crowd-pleaser because many people don't realize how tight they are until they feel this release. By relieving tightness in the perineum floor, this and similar stretches access your Kundalini energy, which resides at the base of your spine and comes to life during orgasm. This stretch also allows you to access your Sacral/Coccyx Love Lock at the point of your perineum and PC muscles (pubococcygeus—the ones you use for Kegel exercises), so practice holding this muscle in contraction and release with that in mind.

1. Stand with your feet a bit more than shoulders' width apart.
2. Engage a pelvic tilt.
3. Try to lift your ribs away from your hips.
4. Slowly lower your torso, and rest your hands on your knees.
5. Try to sink your hips back so that your knees are behind your ankles.
6. Place your hands on the floor and your elbows inside your knees.
7. Flatten your back out like an ironing board.
8. Inhale. As you exhale, sink your torso down as if to bring your navel and sternum down toward the floor.
9. Maintaining a flat back, press your elbows out against your knees. You should feel a stretch in your groin, hamstrings, and pelvic floor.

THIS IS A great time to practice strengthening your PC muscles by contracting them, squeezing as if trying to keep from urinating. Doing these so-called Kegel exercises regularly can improve your orgasmic potential.

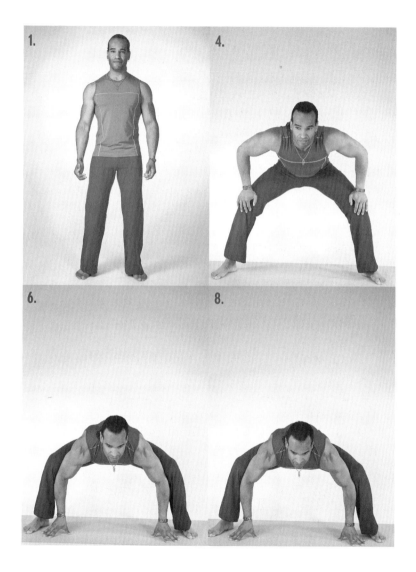

ADDUCTOR (INNER THIGH) STRETCH

HOW TIGHT ARE your inner-thigh muscles normally? Like the Pelvic Perineum Stretch, when these muscles open up, you will feel your groin say, "Oh, yeah!"

1. Perform steps 1 thru 9 from Pelvic Perineum Stretch.
2. Extend your right leg out to the side with your foot pointed straight ahead. Try to press the inside of your right heel into the floor, as if slightly lifting the outer edge of your foot. Your hand and elbow against your left knee will act as a support.
3. Inhale, and extend your right hand out in front of your left foot.
4. Exhale, and sweep your torso and hand over toward your right foot. Slowly feel the stretch in the adductor, the muscle in your inner thigh. You may not be able to reach your foot initially, so practice.
5. Repeat with the other leg.

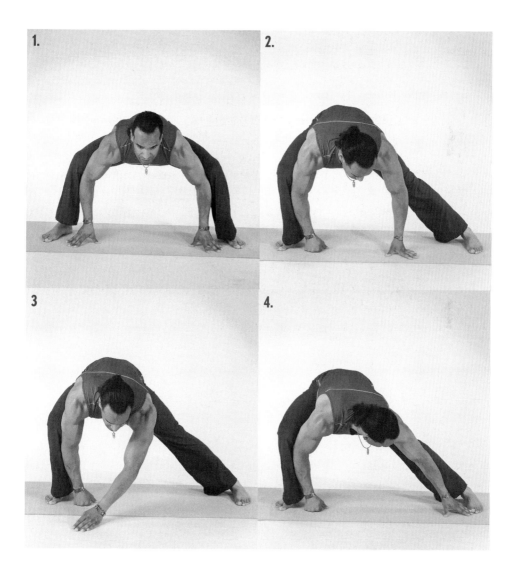

GETTING WARMER:
Partner Stretching

There are lots of benefits to stretching with your partner. First of all, it feels great and will help both of you to relieve a lot of tension and relax. It's something you can share, an excellent way to gain and show appreciation for each other. You will be opening and expanding more than just your physical range of motion, and will get to know each other in new and sometimes surprising ways.

You don't have to be a professional dancer, martial artist, or yoga master to become a great lover! Some of my students still don't dance well but report that they now experience great success in their intimate lives.

THE SUITCASE: SUPER SPINE STRETCH

THIS STRETCH IS a favorite of everyone who learns it, because it really helps release lumbar stress, tension, and pain and allow for greater mobility and range of motion. The Suitcase stretch allows a woman greater ability to lift her legs and more easily present her G-Spot. When a woman lifts her legs it also shortens her vaginal canal, allowing easier access to her cervix. The Suitcase is also a good stretch for a man because it opens his lumbar and improves his ability to maneuver himself to reach the G-spot and other internal areas with a more accurate upward stroke. Finally, the Suitcase is invaluable in preparing your partner's body for the Lumbar Love Lock.

This stretch is quite profound for the recipient. Done gently, it opens up the spine without any effort on their part other than staying relaxed. The levels represent three different areas to be systematically opened in the spine, and should be embarked upon gently as not everyone is flexible enough in the beginning to practice all three levels. Level 1 is a good overall spinal stretch. Level 2 moves more deeply into the lumbar spine and hamstrings. Level 3 is imitative of a partner-assisted Yogic Plow pose, engaging the entire spine in a deep stretch.

Level 1

1. Have your partner lie on their back on the floor, hands down by their sides, pressing their lumbar into the floor.
2. Stand at their feet and have them lift their feet up to you.
3. Have them bend and spread their knees and bring the soles of their feet together, bringing their legs into a diamond shape. (Be sure to bend your own knees to protect your back.) If their back is a little sore or tight, assist them in this motion.

4. Have them inhale. As they exhale, slowly and gently begin moving their heels toward their head, pressing their feet slightly down toward their body. Ask them how they feel as you go, as everyone has a different tolerance and levels of tightness in their lower back and spine.

5. Release and repeat steps 3 and 4.

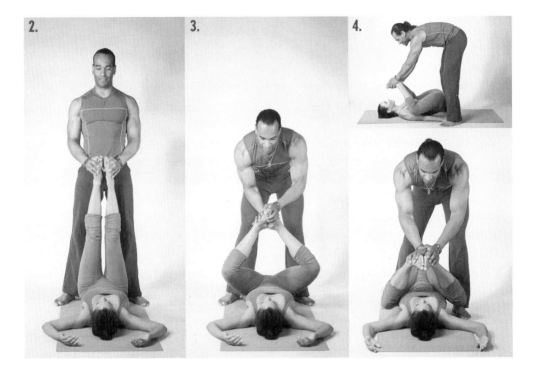

Level 2

1. Kneel beside your partner on the floor. As you press their feet and ankles down with your forearm, press their hamstrings and hips down and back.

2. Proceed with caution. Ask at each point how they feel.

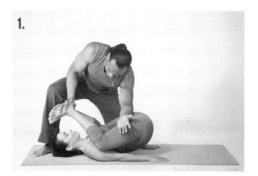

Level 3

1. To further increase the stretch, stand beside your partner and press their heels and ankles down with one hand, guiding their lumbar spine up with your other.

2. You can achieve quite a stretch with this. Your partner's lower back will lift as it stretches. The stretch will eventually reach their neck, having an effect similar to that of a yogic supported Plow Pose.

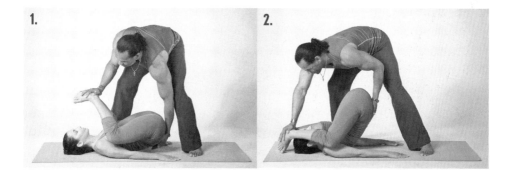

MODIFIED PIGEON

THIS IS A very important stretch, especially for women, because it helps release physical and emotional energy that you may be holding in your hips. Women tend to store a lot of emotional energy in this area, and if it is not released, it can impede their orgasmic potential.

1. Have your partner lay on the floor face up, with their arms by their sides.
2. Kneel down by their left side slightly above their hips (almost at the ribs), as you will stretch their opposite (right) leg first. *Make sure you are stable.*
3. Have them lift their opposite (right) leg up to you.
4. Place the outside of their foot at your waist.
5. Have them inhale. As they exhale, slowly lean your body down to the right toward their chest. (Place your right hand on the floor to support yourself.)
6. Slowly and gently push down with your left hand.
7. Place your right hand on their right knee, and push down gently to increase the stretch. They should feel a stretch in their right hip, glute, and lower back.
8. Repeat the process on the other side.

NOTE: *You are using your body weight to initiate the stretch. Be careful with how much weight and thus pressure you apply. Do not lean all of your weight onto your partner's leg.*

Did you know that massaging the feet is great for arousal, too? The area in the brain that stimulates the sex organs, especially in women, is right next to the area that is stimulated during a foot massage. Experiment and see if you can access that area on your partner!

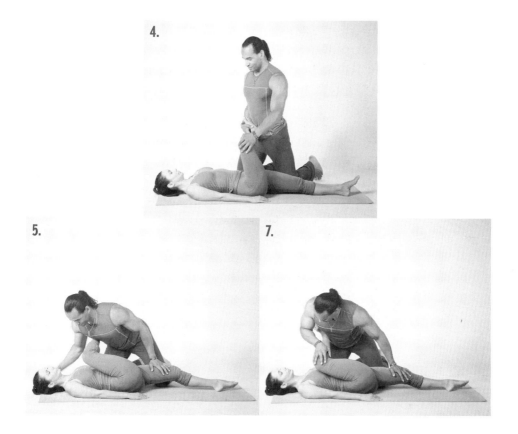

4.

5.

7.

THE BICYCLE

LIKE THE SUITCASE, the Bicycle releases a lot of pent-up lower-back energy and feels incredibly good for the lower back, hips, and spine. It must be done gradually, but it opens up whole new worlds of possibility for both partners to explore. This is a lovely way to loosen up the Lumbar Love Lock literally, laterally, vertically, and horizontally.

1. Have your partner lie on their back, hands down by their sides, pressing their lumbar into the floor.
2. Stand at their feet and have them lift their feet up to you.
3. Hold the soles of their feet.
4. Have them inhale. As they exhale, begin opening their legs, pushing their feet as they bring their knees out to the side.
5. As they feel more open and comfortable, have them inhale again. As they exhale, press their soles and knees down deeper, opening their hips more.
6. Begin pushing the soles of their feet down, first to one side and then to the other, creating a bicycle-pedaling motion.

SEXUALITY WITHOUT SPIRITUALITY leads to vulgarity. Spirituality without sexuality leads to banality. By spirituality I mean consciousness, which to me means paying attention to what really going on. In Tantra the word is *sushumna*, which means to cultivate and assimilate both your consciousness and sex energy.

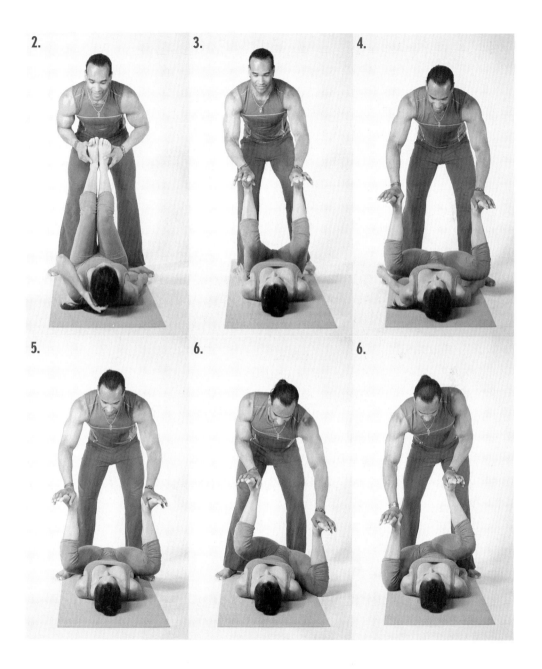

DEEP ADDUCTOR AND GROIN STRETCH

THIS IS A great stretch for opening the groin. It aids maneuverability in both women and men and increases access to a woman's internal and external stimulation points. The more she can open, the easier it is to Mirror and Cue each other, as we will see.

Level 1

1. Have your partner bend and spread their knees and bring the soles of their feet together, bringing their legs into a diamond shape. (Be sure to bend your own knees to protect your back.) If their back is a little sore or tight, assist them in this motion.
2. Kneel beside them on their right side.
3. Place your right hand on their right hip bone and your left hand on their left knee.
4. Have them inhale. As they exhale, pull their right hip toward you as you slowly and gently press their left knee down and forward.

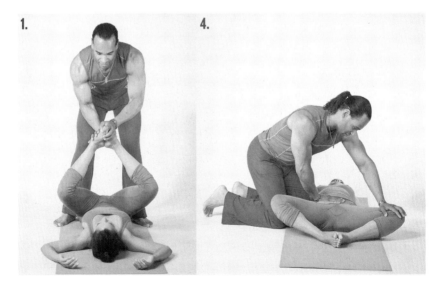

1.   **4.**

Level 2

1. Place your right hand on their right knee and your left hand on their left knee.

2. Have them inhale. As they exhale, begin slowly and gently pressing both knees down and forward.

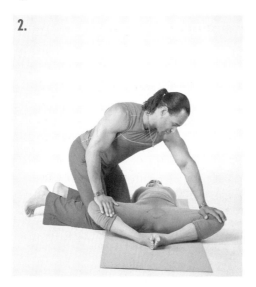

2.

Sexiness is not about age; it's about energy and health. A fit, mature fifty-year-old woman who loves herself is a far better lover than a twenty-five-year-old who thinks she's sexy just because she's "not fat."

TWIST OF FATE FOR TWO

THIS STRETCH REALLY helps your partner release tension from the hips, lower back, and spine. It frees up muscles and energy that help improve performance during side-to-side sexual positions such as spooning. By perfecting this productive pelvic pivot, you can not only prevent sheet burn but also increase the potency of each and every orgasm.

1. Have your partner lie on the floor on their back.
2. Have them bend their left knee up.
3. Kneel down beside the person on their left side, between their arm and bent leg.
4. Gently press their left shoulder down as they rest both arms by their sides.
5. Lift their left leg up until it is perpendicular to the body.
6. Have them move their hips back (right hip down, left up) so their hip is back and in line with their head.
7. Have them inhale. As they exhale, still pressing their left shoulder toward the floor, gently press their left knee down toward the floor.
8. Repeat on the other side.

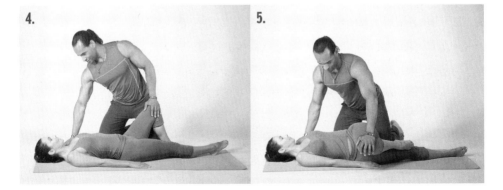

LEG-OVER TWIST OF FATE FOR TWO

SIMILAR TO THE Twist of Fate for Two, this stretch goes deeper into the hip musculature, allowing more sensual mobility by freeing up the more-intricate hip muscles for service.

1. Repeat steps 1 through 6 of Twist of Fate for Two.
2. This time, have them put their right knee over their left knee.
3. Press down gently as they exhale.
4. Repeat on the other side.

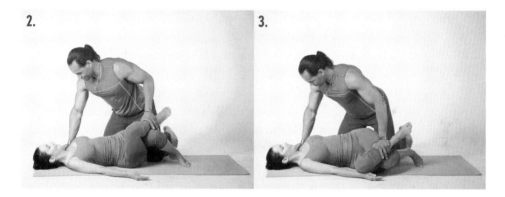

THE TWIST OF Fate for Two stretches are great for increasing your overall range of motion and relieving pain, but they are essential for releasing energy and improving the hip mobility you need for full enjoyment of intimate activities. They even may save you a trip to the chiropractor.

LEG-UNDER TWIST OF FATE FOR TWO

THIS ONE FREES up more torso and hip muscles for greater hip articulation, which you'll appreciate when the time comes!

1. Repeat steps 1 thru 6 from the Twist of Fate for Two.
2. This time, have them put their right knee under their left knee.
3. Have them inhale. As they exhale, still pressing their left shoulder toward the floor, gently press their left knee down toward the floor.
4. Repeat on the other side.

As they are moving their knee over, try to keep their left shoulder down, as it may come up off the floor. Don't force it back down, and don't force the knee if your partner can't push it very far. Ask your partner how their hip and back feel before continuing, and proceed carefully if they feel all right. Be sure to get into a firmly rooted and supported position yourself so you do not rock forward, backward, or side to side.

As you hold their left arm or near the floor, be sure to have them inhale. As they exhale, gently move their left knee down toward the floor. Continue to monitor them constantly, asking how they're feeling. Release and repeat this last step a few times before switching legs.

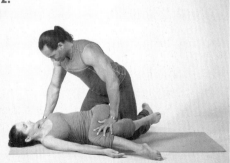

2.

FACEDOWN TWIST OF FATE FOR TWO

THIS ALLOWS YOUR lover to relax as they prepare their body either for massage or an adventurous evening. Either way, they'll be grateful to you for the way this makes them feel.

1. Have your partner lie down on their right side, with the right arm stretched out in back of them. Have them rest their left arm in front of them. You may want to put a folded towel or pillow beneath their head.
2. Have them lift their right (bottom) leg up, perpendicular to their body, and bend their knee to a ninety-degree angle.
3. Have them reach their left arm out across in front of them.
4. Kneel in back of them, your left knee near the small of their back.
5. Have them inhale. As they exhale, press down and in with your palm, slowly and gently moving their shoulder toward the floor. They should feel a nice stretch in their back and spine.
6. Gently massage your partner's back and side.
7. Repeat step 5, 6, and 7 as needed.
8. Repeat on their other side.

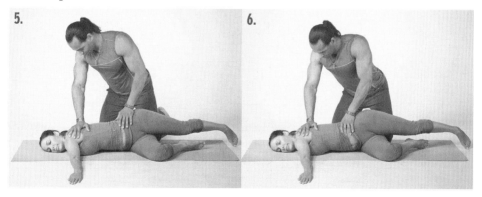

LEG-OVER, FACEDOWN
TWIST OF FATE FOR TWO

LIKE THE OTHER variations on the Twist of Fate for Two, this one adds another tantalizing twist to a delicious stretch that will leave your partner's back, hips, and spine feeling alive, relaxed and, if need be, very, very ready.

1. Have your partner lie down on their right side, with the right arm stretched out in back of them. Have them rest their left arm in front of them. You may want to put a folded towel or pillow beneath their head.
2. Have them lift their right (bottom) leg up, perpendicular to their body, and bend their knee to a ninety-degree angle.
3. Have them reach their left arm out across in front of them.
4. Kneel in back of them, your left knee near the small of their back.
5. Have them inhale. As they exhale, press down and in with your palm, slowly and gently moving their shoulder toward the floor. They should feel a nice stretch in their back and spine.
6. Now have them put their left leg under their right leg to increase the stretch.
7. Have them inhale. As they exhale, press down and in with your palm, slowly and gently moving their shoulder toward the floor.
8. Gently massage your partner's back and spine.
9. For an extra stretch, you can also pull back on their hips as you push down on their shoulders.

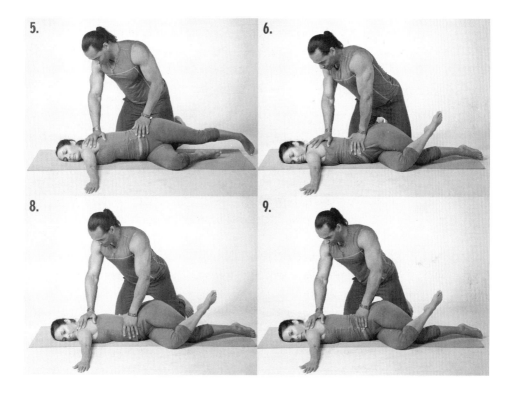

5.

6.

8.

9.

PARTNER-ASSISTED TRANSVERSE TWIST

THIS IS A nice adjustment aid that can be done anytime and anywhere to help your partner loosen up his or her back and spine. It feels really nice to receive this from a lover.

1. Begin with your partner's shoulders squared, knees bent, and arms up and out to the sides.
2. Stand in front of your partner, slightly to their left. Step your right foot across in front of your partner's left, and have them engage in a pelvic tilt. (Engage in one yourself while you are at it.)
3. Straighten your partner's spine by lifting their ribs up and away from their hips.
4. Place the outside of your right knee against the inside of their left knee.
5. Place your right hand under their right shoulder, firmly cupping the front of the shoulder. Then place your left hand against the back of their left shoulder.
6. Have them inhale. As they exhale, gently push their left shoulder forward while pulling their right shoulder back. They should feel a stretch in their back, hip, and spine.
7. Repeat on the opposite side.

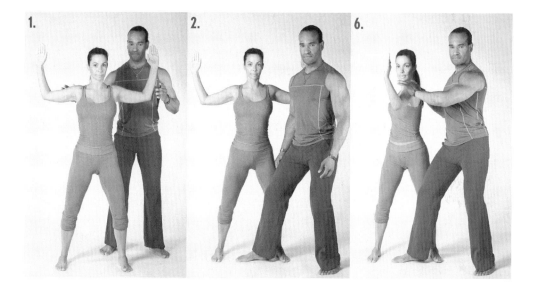

1.

2.

6.

STICKING WITH IT

$\mathcal{W}$E BECOME WHAT we practice most. One way or another, we all become a master of something. Every day we train our brain to be a certain way, to think a certain way, and we train ourselves to feel, react, and respond a certain way. If we work out mindlessly in order to get it over with, or to avoid the pain, we are also training ourselves to miss the pleasure of stretching and conditioning our body. There is a Chinese symbol called Ren, which means "human being." It also means perseverance. The symbol is a knife above a heart, which means that even with a knife held over your heart, you persist and persevere. The point I'm trying to make is that—you guessed it—in order to become a real human being, we all have to go through some pain. And in order to become a great lover, we need to be willing to go through some uncomfortable or scary moments, especially when we see ourselves in the mirror of a relationship.

When you "ride the burn" of the resistance while exercising, several things are happening simultaneously. You may think you are just training a muscle, but you are really training your brain, your heart, and your spirit. You are teaching yourself to embrace rather than escape adversity. You are teaching yourself to be a warrior in both life and love. Remember, where there is no physical or mental adversity, there will be atrophy. And one who cannot endure pain cannot bring pleasure.

In Tantra, learning to "ride the wave" means learning to delay sexual gratification. To withhold pleasure is another way of saying that you are able to withstand pain. If you can learn to do this, to breathe it up, you can train your lower energy for a higher purpose. You can turn your coal into a diamond. Building up a muscle and building up an orgasm are not terribly different processes; if you have the passion, the spirit, and the heart, it will show in both the bedroom and the weight room. If you can learn to "ride the burn," you will build a great body. If you can learn to "ride the wave," you will come to new levels of awareness and build up your orgasmic energy for a more powerful and fulfilling release.

Now that you've limbered up, it's time to start practicing the exercises that will condition you to do the positions. Being able to move is one thing, but being able to keep moving is quite another. Remember that we're aiming for progress, not perfection, so find what works for you, make it fun, and stick with it. The long- and short-term benefits are worth it! You won't run out of steam in the bedroom, and you will be better equipped to use the steam that you have. You will feel more alive and feed your passion for life. The word *passion* is derived from the Latin word *passio*, which means "suffering being acted upon." Embrace the burn and become your most passionate self!

HEATING UP:
Strengthening Exercises

The body of the Corvette Stingray from 1968 to 1973 has one of the sexiest automobile shapes ever created, because it mimics the female shape. Those Corvettes looked as if they had a corset: The front fenders flare and the rear quarters, like hips, have heavenly humps that hug some hefty tires. Our bodies also come factory-equipped with an internal corset called the transverse abdominus, which wraps around your torso below your ribs (fig. 20). Strengthen your transverse abs, along with your lower abs and obliques, and your hips will hug those curves.

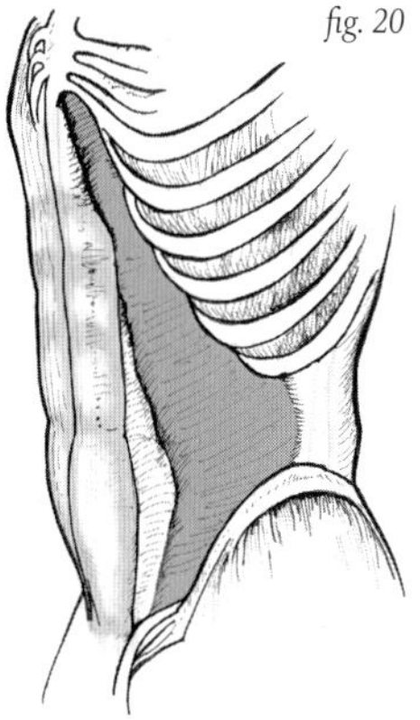

fig. 20

BAD KITTY

WHEN YOU'RE GRINDING out this smoldering tricep exercise, picture being down on all fours with Joe Cocker's classic song "You Can Leave Your Hat On" blaring. At the climactic point in a song you bust out the exotic dancer "hair flip" move, followed by a wink and a hand slap to the floor. The women in my classes didn't stop at that. No, they proceed to add meows and "tail wagging," and lots of it. The next class they said, "Make sure we save time for the Bad Kitty!"

1. Put on some music that inspires you.
2. Kneel down on the floor.
3. Create a square with your hands beneath your shoulders, knees beneath your hips.
4. Engage a pelvic tilt.
5. Inhale, and lean your shoulders down slightly over your hands.
6. Lean your shoulders down and forward. As you exhale, use your triceps to push straight up, keeping your shoulders in front of your hands.
7. Push straight back up three-quarters of the way toward neutral (but don't rest!).
8. Repeat until the song is over.

> FOR ALL BAD Kitties, always engage a pelvic tilt and do not lock your arms. To work your pectorals more, spread your fingers out wider. Always keep your shoulders in front of your hands.

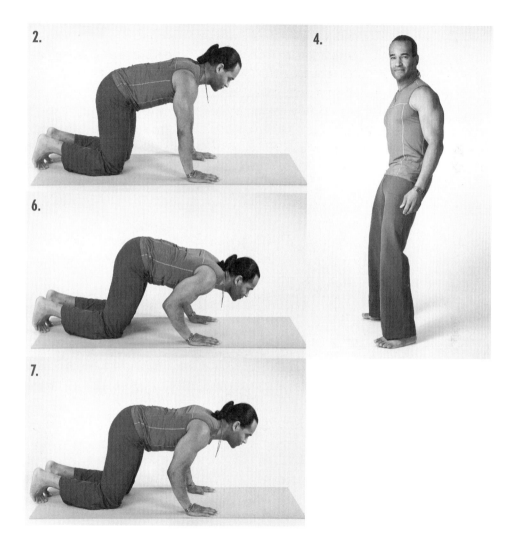

BAD KITTY CAT ROLL

1. Kneel down on the floor.
2. Create a square with your hands beneath your shoulders, knees beneath your hips.
3. Engage a pelvic tilt.
4. Inhale, and lean your shoulders down slightly over your hands.
5. Roll your body down, forward, up and around.
6. Now try rolling both forward and backward.

According to Dr. Laura Berman in *Real Sex for Real Women*, experiencing an orgasm during a loving sexual encounter at least three times a week can help you to look seven to twelve years younger.

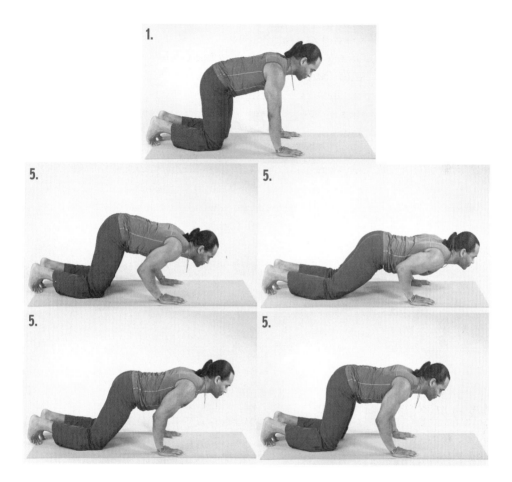

BAD CATWALK

1. Kneel down on the floor.
2. Create a square with your hands beneath your shoulders, knees beneath your hips.
3. Engage a pelvic tilt.
4. Inhale, and lean your shoulders down slightly over your hands.
5. Support yourself with one arm while you extend the other arm forward, stretching passionately with your hand in a claw shape, switching hands to the beat. This is a classic stripper being a cat move, so if you are a man and you practice this exercise you get extra credit!

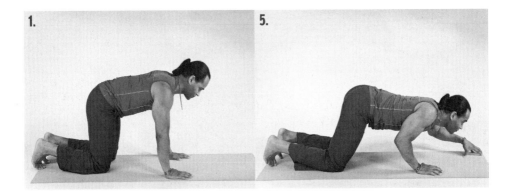

BAD CAT KICKBACK

1. Kneel down on the floor.
2. Create a square with your hands beneath your shoulders, knees beneath your hips.
3. Engage a pelvic tilt.
4. Inhale, and lean your shoulders down slightly over your hands.
5. Lean down so that your left ear is just above the floor, and bring your right knee to your elbow.
6. Inhale. As you exhale, push up and extend your right leg back with either flexed or pointed foot.
7. Repeat until fatigued. Then try the same thing on your other side.

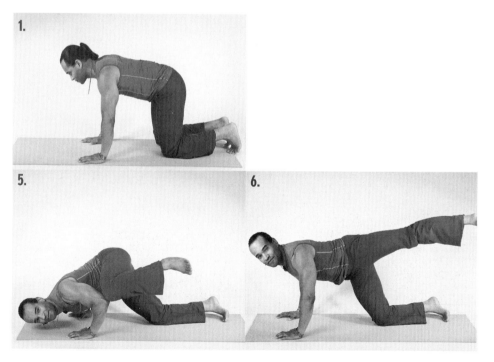

CORE OF LOVE (AB TRAINING)

WHEN DOING ABDOMINAL exercises of any kind, *never* sit or rock on your tailbone. Your tailbone/sacrum/coccyx is the origin of your Kundalini (sex energy). Yogis once attempted to kill off their sex drive by rocking on their tailbones. This is not our goal. Your tailbone is your trigger to send orgasmic energy up your spine.

1. Sit on the floor with your knees together and bent at a forty-five-degree angle.
2. Leaning back on your elbows for support, engage a pelvic tilt.
3. Keeping your shoulders back, place one open hand, and then the other, over your knees.
4. Inhale, and then roll back until your fingertips are over your knees.
5. Exhale and move forward until your palms are back over your knees.
6. Repeat steps 4 and 5 for three sets, each time until fatigued. Try to *feel* the burn just a little longer each time!

NOTE: *If you are just starting out or if you have back issues, try the same exercise using a ball or a rolled mat placed at your lumbar spine. This will help give overall ab strength to help you "go the distance."*

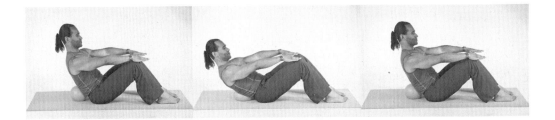

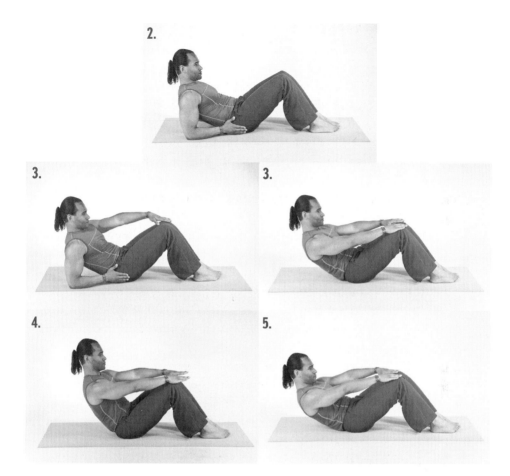

During ab exercises, imagine that you're trying to keep the label on the inside back of your pants stuck to the floor. This should help you keep your hips and navel stationary. In all of the ab exercises, make it a point to practice pulling your navel toward your pubic bone.

ARCHER ABS

DID YOU KNOW that Cupid and Eros are the Roman and Greek versions of the same winged deity? They may differ in their approach, but they're both aiming at the heart!

Try this to music!

1. Sit on the floor with your knees bent.
2. Leaning back on your elbows for support, engage a pelvic tilt.
3. Keeping your shoulders back, place one open hand and then the other over your knees.
4. Exhaling, slowly roll your back down until your fingertips are over your knees.
5. As you lean back, turn to one side and pretending you are holding a bow and arrow, pull your arm back as if to fire an arrow.
6. Come forward and bring your hands over your knees again, or together in front of you.
7. Repeat on the other side. Continue for as long as you can.

FRANK ZANE, WHO won three consecutive Mr. Olympia titles from 1977 to 1979, had what many feel was the best natural-looking physique in bodybuilding history. He said, "Train the lower abs and the upper abs will take care of themselves." This is a profound insight for anyone who wants to do well in the weight room or, for our purposes, the bedroom.

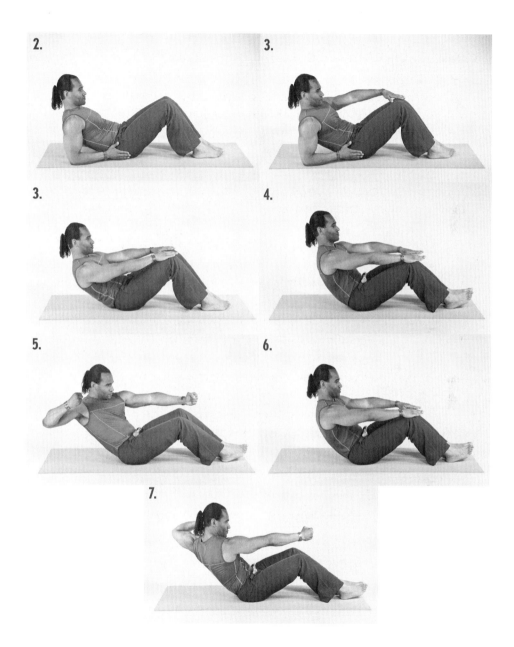

2.

3.

3.

4.

5.

6.

7.

ROCK THE BOAT

ASIDE FROM BEING incredibly fun to do, Rock the Boat rocks your oblique and transverse abs all at once. This is like paddling a canoe—first left, then right, and so on. Make it a sensual flowing movement as if to really *feeeeel* the water. Grind this one out to one of your favorite tunes and indulge in the sexy twisting and turning motion. This exercise will get you ready to move from the mat to the mattress in a hurry as you heat up your core.

1. Sit on the floor with your knees bent.
2. Leaning back on your elbows for support, engage a pelvic tilt.
3. Keeping your shoulders back, place one open hand and then the other over your knees.
4. Keeping your shoulders back, place your open hands over your knees.
5. As you exhale, slowly roll your back down so your fingertips are over your knees.
6. Pretending you are holding a canoe paddle, twist your body to the left and paddle on one beat of the music, then twist to the right on the next beat. As you paddle to one side, lean your knees to the opposite side.
7. Repeat until fatigued.

ANY TIME YOU are exercising your transverse abs, as in Rock the Boat or Archer Abs, always think of moving your hips toward the opposite shoulder. For instance, when you are rowing in Rock the Boat, when your left shoulder moves toward the centerline, visualize twisting and moving the top of your right hip toward your centerline.

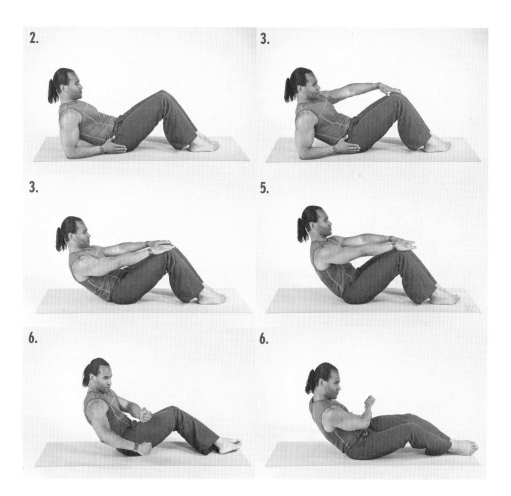

HIP LIFT (LOWER ABS)

IF THIS EXERCISE is difficult, try putting a pillow or a folded towel beneath your sacrum. This is one of the best ways to tone your lower abs and eventually perfect the motion of the ocean. This movement will not only help you to strengthen and define your lower abs but, once you get it down, to move like Michael and shake it like Shakira!

1. Lie on the floor and bend your knees up to a ninety-degree angle (forming an upside-down L). Your shins should be horizontal.
2. Brace your hands flat on the floor beside you, palms down.
3. Inhale. As you exhale, lift your knees toward the ceiling by raising your tailbone/sacrum off the floor, trying not to use momentum.
4. Slowly lower them back down.
5. Repeat until fatigued.

Typical gym ab exercises, where you change your hip-to-leg angle by moving your legs—such as bicycling, leg lifts, Roman chair crunches, reverse curls, or hanging leg or knee lifts—often diminish their intended effectiveness by using the hip flexors as the primary muscle group, instead of the lower abs (the core) that we are focusing on.

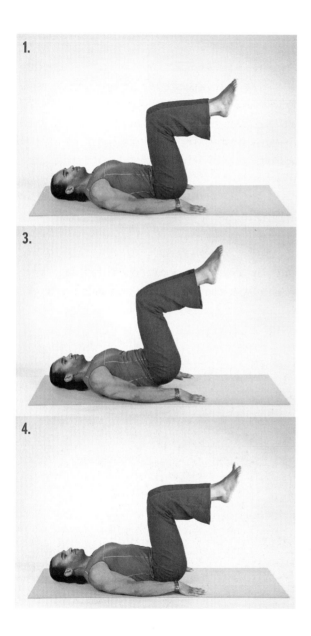

THE FROG

BET YOU DIDN'T realize your biology class would aid you in other ways! This lower-ab strengthener helps you articulate and practice movements that will immediately make you a better lover. The frog is a Lumbar Love Lock facilitator that will help men smoothly and comfortably transition from coital position to position without losing contact and continuity with his lover's internal pleasure points.

1. Sit on the floor with your knees bent.
2. Leaning on your elbows for support, engage a pelvic tilt. Again, pretend you're trying to keep your pants label pressed to the floor so that you don't move your hips or navel. Although it is not necessary, you can place a small weight on your lower abs to keep from using your hip flexors.
3. Bring the soles of your feet together while maintaining a pelvic tilt. When you do this, creating a diamond with your knees apart, you are better isolating your lower abs by taking your hip flexors out of the equation.
4. Inhale. As you exhale, begin contracting your lower abdominals by curling your hips up.
5. Slowly lift your feet and legs by lifting your pubic bone and sacrum off the floor. Try not to use your hip flexors.
6. Lower slowly, without touching the floor again.
7. Repeat until fatigued.

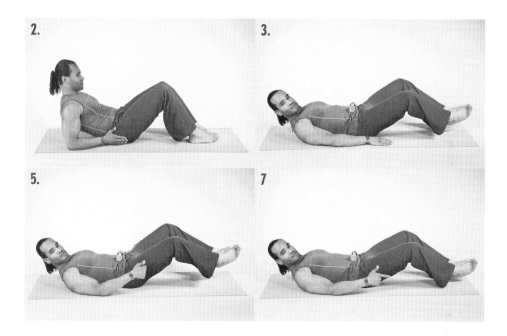

NOTE: *If you find it difficult to place your feet in a low position, try holding them up a little higher.*

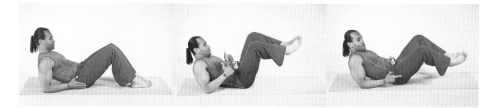

THE FROG ARTIST

WHEN YOU FEEL comfortable with The Frog, try the Frog Artist—it's a coordinating articulation exercise that brings in more hip articulations, training you to shift and move your hips from side to side. It's amazing for strengthening your abs. Each sweet stroke will help you make a masterpiece of every erotic encounter.

1. Sit on the floor with your knees bent.

2. Leaning back on your elbows for support, engage a pelvic tilt. Again, pretend you're trying to keep your pants tag pressed to the floor so that you don't move your hips or navel.

3. Bring the soles of your feet together while maintaining a pelvic tilt.

4. Visualize holding a pen between the soles of your feet.

5. With that imaginary pen, try drawing circles, ovals, squares, rectangles, and triangles.

6. Practice writing your name or spelling out words until your abs run out of things to say!

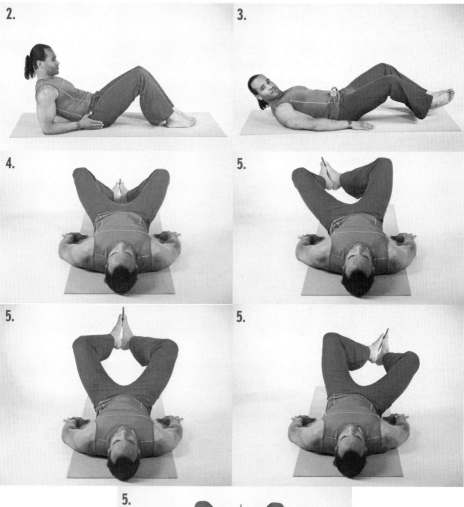

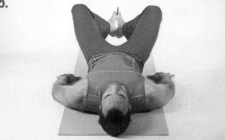

ROCK THE PLANK

THE PLANK IS an advanced exercise traditionally done in yoga. I will show you how to Rock the Plank from a modified traditional plank and from your knees (see "Rock the Plank from Your Knees," below), in the event that you need to work up to it. (If this is your first time trying the plank, or if you have lower back or abdominal issues, you might want to try it from your knees first.) Rock the Plank is a Lumbar Lock that will keep you a prisoner of pleasure through wave after wave of orgasm: strong lower abs and a pelvic rocking motion that will allow you a Deep Press (page 140) that will push and hold all the right buttons. Guys, you'll often find yourselves in this position, so practice it!

1. Lie on the floor on your stomach and press your knees into the floor, about three inches apart.
2. Straighten your legs, lifting your knees off the floor by pressing your toes into the floor. You are now in a forward pelvic tilt, engaging your core, and supporting yourself in a plank on your elbows and feet.
3. Root your toes firmly into the floor. Engage a pelvic tilt.
4. Lift yourself up to a plank position by propping up your torso, bringing your elbows beneath your shoulders, and placing your palms down. Try to keep a flat upper back; do not arch it up like a cat.
5. Maintaining your pelvic tilt, inhale. As you exhale, contract your lower abs to create a more pronounced pelvic tilt.
6. Inhale and release to a neutral position (with your pelvic tilt still engaged). While rocking or holding the plank, *never* allow your lumbar spine to sway back.
7. Exhale, and engage another exaggerated pelvic tilt by contracting your lower abs.

8. Repeat as many times as you can.

9. If you want to strengthen your core even further, try extending a hand out to one side, then switch hands to support yourself on the other elbow and extend the other hand.

DID YOU KNOW that the first vibrator was sold by Sears & Roebuck in the 1800s for "medical" purposes? Boys may have their toys in the garage, but girls keep theirs in the closet. Guys, all those shoeboxes—decoys!

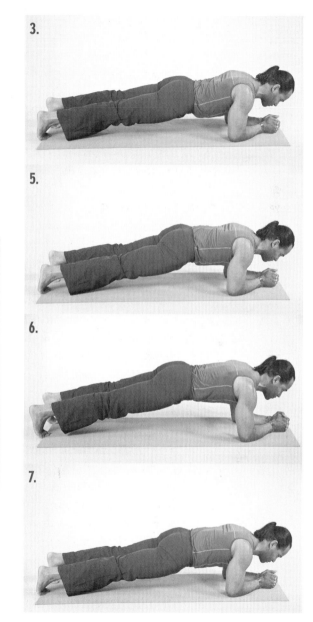

3.

5.

6.

7.

ROCK THE PLANK FROM YOUR KNEES

THIS MODIFIED ROCKING of the plank from your knees rocks worlds as well! Holding the contracted plank from your knees is a very effective core exercise, especially for beginners.

1. Lie facedown on the floor.
2. Press your knees into the floor about three to six inches apart.
3. Engage your core, creating a forward pelvic tilt, and press your elbows into the floor shoulders' width apart, directly under your shoulders with your palms facing down. See how well you can support yourself there.
4. Exhale, and try contracting your lower abs while moving into a deep pelvic tilt forward. Remember to try to move your pubic bone toward your navel.
5. Release the pelvic tilt slightly as you inhale, moving to a slight forward pelvic tilt.
6. Exhale and contract your lower abs again, moving into a deep pelvic tilt forward. *Be sure that you do not have an arched cat's back. You want your back flat—like a plank!*
7. Inhale. As you exhale, move again into a deep pelvic tilt.
8. After you have successfully accomplished this and feel you can do a sufficient number of repetitions without feeling any strain on your lower back, wait a while and then try a straightforward Rock the Plank (page 108).

3.

4.

5.

7.

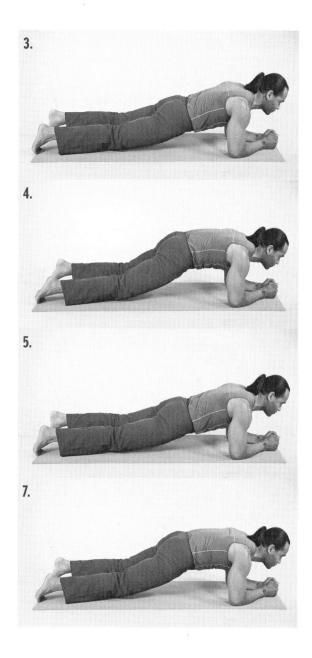

HIP LIFT

WHEN DONE CORRECTLY, this is one of the best lower-ab exercises out there. The Hip Lift will keep your Hip Drop (page 132) hot and heavy and pave the way for the Lumbar Love Lock.

1. Lie on your back with your lumbar planted firmly on the floor.
2. Place your palms down on the floor, preparing to use them as a brace.
3. Bend your knees to a ninety-degree angle with your shins horizontal.
4. Inhale. As you exhale, try to lift your hips off the floor as if trying to curl your sacrum up, lifting your knees straight up off the floor.
5. *Slowly* lower yourself back down. Try not to use momentum up or down. If this is too difficult, try putting a pillow or rolled-up mat underneath your hips.

Remember: You want to *im*prove, not prove! Go at your own pace and have fun.

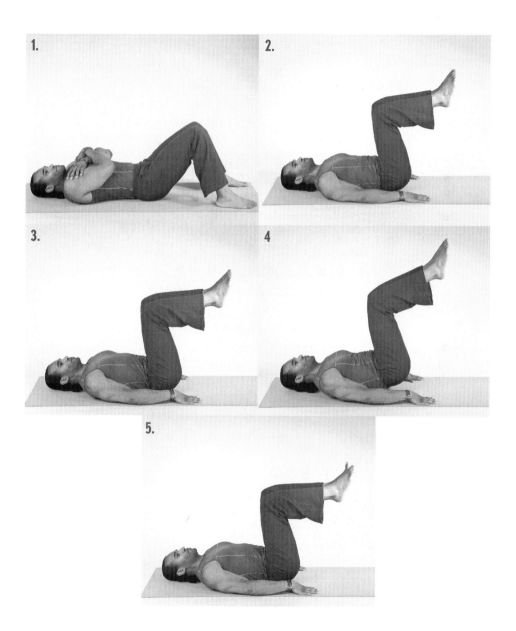

FROG HIP SHIFT

TRY A SLIGHTLY more advanced move for your obliques and transverse abdominals. The Frog Hip Shift will shift you into new realms of satisfaction by strengthening your side-to-side movement, making every angle the right angle.

1. Sit on the floor with your knees bent.

2. Leaning back on your elbows for support, engage a pelvic tilt. Pretend you're trying to keep your pants label pressed to the floor so that you don't move your hips or navel.

3. Bring the soles of your feet together while maintaining a pelvic tilt.

4. Inhale. As you exhale, begin contracting your lower abdominals by curling your hips up.

5. Slowly lift your feet and legs by lifting your pubic bone and sacrum off the floor. Try not to use your hip flexors to lift your feet.

6. Rotate your waist, and shift your hips back and forth.

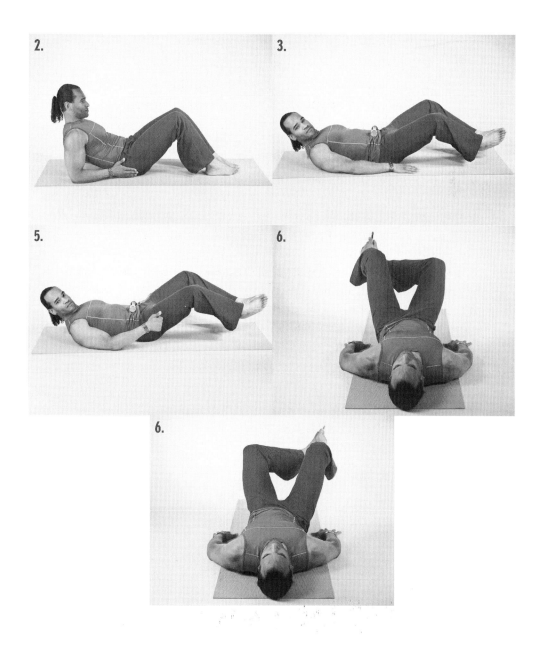

HIP SHIFT (LOWER ABS, OBLIQUES. AND TRANSVERSE ABS)

THE MOTION OF the ocean catches some waves here!

1. Lay on your back with your lumbar planted firmly on the floor.
2. Place your hands palms down on the floor, using them as a brace.
3. Bend your knees to a ninety-degree angle, with your shins horizontal.
4. Inhale. As you exhale try to lift your hips off the floor as if trying to curl your sacrum up, lifting your knees straight up off the floor.
5. Exhale and lift your sacrum off the floor, tilting your knees to your right.
6. *Slowly* lower yourself back down.
7. Now try lifting to your left. Try not to use momentum. If this is too difficult, try putting a pillow or rolled-up mat underneath your hips.

Once you've effectively trained your transverse abs and obliques, you will be better able to cue up and tune in to your lover's hot spots. These moves will also help eliminate your love handles!

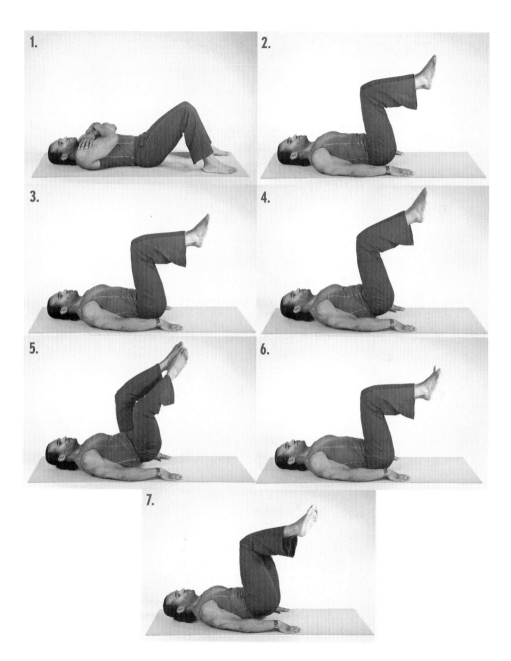

REACHING FOR GRAPES

THIS ONE STRENGTHENS your obliques. You'll have some sexy sidewinder motions when you're done with these, not to mention a smaller waistline.

1. Lay on your right side, resting your elbow slightly underneath and in front of your head, pressing your right hand down on the floor.
2. Bend your left leg up, placing your left foot on the floor in front of your right leg with your right leg straight out and down. Lift your right arm up, as if reaching for grapes in an ancient Roman or Greek picture.
3. Try to lift your left shoulder off the floor.
4. Lower your shoulder without putting it back down completely. You should feel your oblique muscles engage on your lower left side.
5. Do as many repetitions as you can, then switch sides. Do three sets on each side.

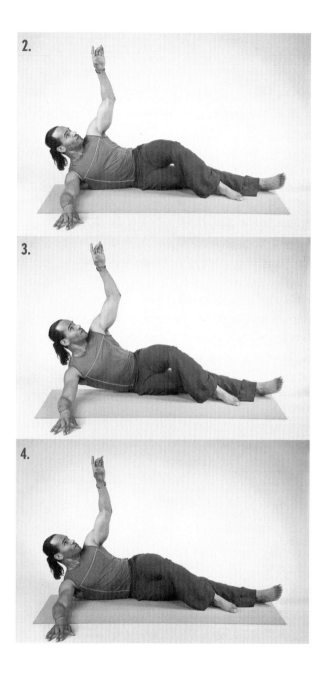

ILIAC LIFT (STANDING OBLIQUES)

YOU WILL GAIN balance and lateral articulation from this hip bone lift, adding a side scoop motion to your repertoire.

1. Stand with your feet a bit more than shoulders' width apart.

2. Engage a pelvic tilt.

3. Leaning to your right, sink down a little so your right hip is over your right heel, and extend your left leg and foot out slightly to the side. Your navel should be over your right foot.

4. Raise both hands above your head.

5. Inhale. As you exhale, engage your obliques, the muscles on your side between your waist and your hips, and try to lift your right hip (iliac bone) up toward your right rib. This should cause your right foot to lift off the floor.

6. Lower your hip and foot, allowing your foot to slightly touch the floor.

7. Repeat until slightly fatigued; then try the other side.

8. Do three sets on each side.

IN *THE SECRETS of the Super Young*, Dr. David Weeks writes that improving the quality of your sex life can make you look four to seven years younger, if not more. Vigorous sex can release small bursts of human growth hormone into your system up to seven times a day, improving lean body mass and reducing fatty tissue.

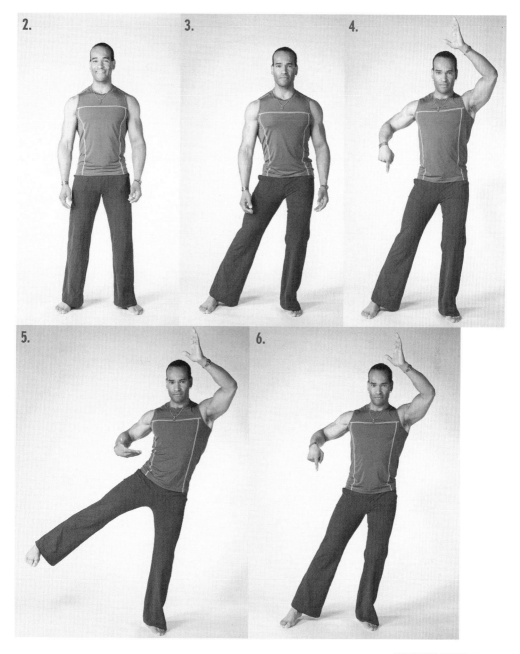

HIP LIFT (OBLIQUES)

HERE YOUR OBLIQUES are engaged along with your lower abs to help you attain supremely sexy pelvic power. This side-to-side shifting motion will get attention in the gym and results in the bedroom.

1. Lie on the floor and bend your knees at a ninety-degree angle so that your shins are horizontal.

2. Place your hands flat on the floor beside you, palms down.

3. As you lift your hips up, twist your knees to the right.

4. Drop your hips and knees down slowly to the center.

5. Then lift them to the left.

6. Repeat until fatigued.

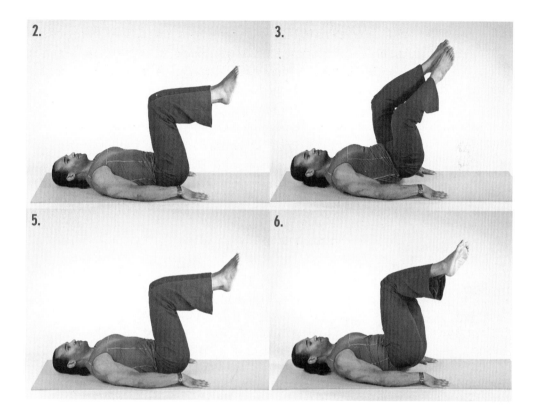

SOLE LIFT (ADDUCTOR)

YOU'LL FEEL THIS one deep into your groin. People often smile while doing the Sole Lift because they notice that when they start to feel fatigue, a peculiar sensation can set in. Because working the deep groin muscles, especially those in the pelvic floor and lower abs, also work our genitals, you may sometimes feel a bit sexually aroused during these routines. The adductor muscle in this position is left to itself to lift the legs up and down. It is supported and rooted in the pelvic and perineal muscles. Women and men alike can feel a surprisingly pleasing sensation when they hold their legs close and pull their knees together.

1. Lie on the floor on your side. Lean on your elbow.
2. Extend your bottom leg so it is perpendicular to your body.
3. Lift your top leg and bend your knee, pressing the foot of your top leg firmly to the floor to provide support.
4. Place your top hand on the floor between your legs for more support and stability.
5. Engage your lower abdominals and core.
6. Exhale, then lift the extended leg up.
7. Inhale while lowering it down.
8. Practice making small circles without lowering your foot back to the floor.

2.

6.

7.

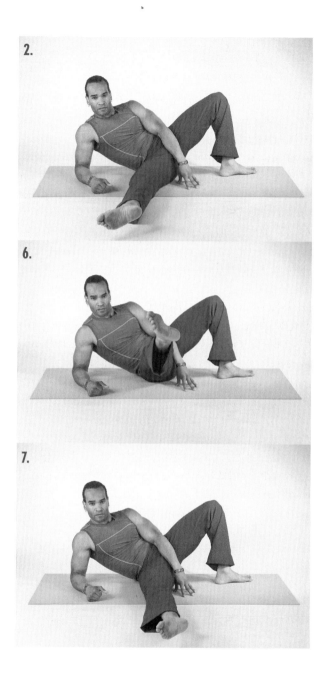

PELVIC PERINEUM STRETCH (UPPER REAR HAMSTRINGS AND QUADS)

WELCOME TO YOUR body once again! You might notice a significant amount of heat being released in this position: Kundalini energy from the base of your spine. Strengthening the perineum floor and PC muscles improves both the sex act itself and the intensity and potency of your orgasms. This exercise is especially helpful for women who want to tone up the hard-to-reach saddlebag area, where the hamstrings (backs of the legs) meet the glutes (derrière). The truth is, for both women and men, this area plays an important role in the articulation of the pelvis during lovemaking. It also works the quads, which are the body's number-one calorie and fat burner. It tightens, tones, and adds great shape to the glutes, giving great definition and lift to the lower glute area.

1. Stand with your feet a bit more than shoulders' width apart.
2. Engage a pelvic tilt. Try to lift your ribs away from your hips.
3. Slowly lower your torso until your elbows rest on your knees. Try to sink your hips back so that your knees are behind your ankles.
4. Place your hands on the floor inside your feet, with your elbows inside your knees.
5. Flatten your back out like an ironing board.
6. Inhale. As you exhale, sink your torso as if to bring your navel and sternum down toward the floor. Now is a good time to strengthen your PC muscles by squeezing them as if trying to keep from urinating. Exhale and hold the semi-squatting position—your back flat, your navel toward your spine—for ten seconds as you tense up and contract your PC muscles, then release.

7. Place your hands on your knees, inhale, and sink your hips down.

8. Exhale and raise your hips up without straightening your legs.

9. Practice going down (inhaling) and up (exhaling) until fatigued. Try doing a few more than you think you can.

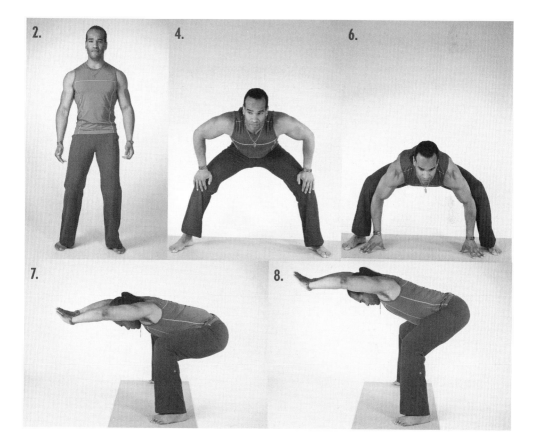

By stretching and strengthening the groin muscles, we are also tapping into and releasing Kundalini energy. My students describe this experience as a rush of heat up their spine. This is caused by the pulling on the many muscles attached to the coccyx (tailbone), including the PC or pubococcygeus muscle. In both sexes, the PC muscle is a hammocklike muscle that stretches from the pubic bone to the coccyx, forming the floor of the pelvic cavity and supporting the pelvic organs. The muscles that stretch across the perineum floor play a profound part in the potency of your orgasm, so, by strengthening them, you're literally getting to the roots of sexual rapture.

BEFORE PLAY

*g*ROWING UP, I was the only black kid in the history of the world who had no rhythm. I mean none. I could *not* dance. It wasn't until junior high, when I was asked to dance by a girl I had a crush on, and had to watch her dance with a friend of mine instead, that I was crushed by not being able to dance. I had only one hope—*Soul Train*. I stayed home when my friends went out and practiced relentlessly. I began to see that dance and kung fu had a lot of the same movements. (I later found out Bruce Lee had been the cha-cha champion of Hong Kong!) I got good at popping, locking, waving, and boogaloo. When my mom died before my senior year of high school, I sank myself into my dance practice even more. It became an emotional release for me.

Later, I ended up dating a fantastic girl who was a jazz/modern and tap dancer. Her family of musicians kind of adopted me. I revamped my dance style and thought I was pretty good—until I met the Nunez sisters. These girls took movement to a whole new level; they were like super Latin dance queens. In dancing with them I learned how to move my hips in ways that shy gear heads from Boston like me just didn't do. People told me I made Michael Jackson look bad. I learned to mirror and move in sync with a woman and found myself dancing for hours straight in the clubs. I also noticed that, now that I could dance, I was the one getting asked. I hardly ever had to ask anyone.

At one point I had an opportunity to perform in some clubs in Japan, and I took it. When I got there and they saw me dance, I was asked if I would consider working as a stripper, and teaching some of the other erotic dancers my moves. Hesitantly, I agreed, but would only go down to a Speedo. I taught the guys some movements and did the show, but since I wasn't stripping down all the way, I had to find other ways to spice up my shows. I began bringing the women up on stage, laying them down, and feeding them exotic fruits dripping with honey. Sometimes I would do a scene similar to the one in the movie *Ghost*: Holding their hands from behind, we would squeeze the honey onto the fruit together. I began to notice that the response I was getting was different than that of the typical stripper show—it was deeper. I got more tips, but also more requests to "table talk." Yes, table talk! The women wanted me to dance with and for them, but more than anything, they wanted to talk with me. They told me they liked my romantic approach to performance. They liked that my shows took them out of themselves. They imagined things. And they expressed all this to me all in Japan-glish! At every show I heard screams of "Billy, I love you!" I was on to something.

Later, when I returned to the States, I began to train Chippendale dancers while I continued to dance in clubs, private home shows, and bachelorette parties. I kept up with my romantic themes, always asking the women during and after the show what they liked and why. Why were they there? What were they looking for that they weren't getting at home? It got to the point where my shows had developed kind of a cult following. I would be in a supermarket and women would come up and say, "You're the 'Kiss from a Rose' Seal guy" or "You're the 'No Ordinary Love' Sade guy!" They would put money in my belt right then and there. I even had one woman scream out in the middle of a crowded mall, while I was doing my day job demonstrating a Health Rider during the Christmas rush, "Wooo, ride' em, cowboy! I'd know those hip moves anywhere. You're the stripper guy from the Palace. Here's a gift for you." And she proceeded to tip me right there in the mall, in front of everyone, while I rode the Health Rider.

More important and useful than what she shoved in my belt was what she put in my mind. Bottom line? Women *love* guys who can move. So, fellas, shall we dance?

YOU MAY USE your legs to stabilize yourself during sex, but sexual precision is all about your hips, which are controlled by your core. This is why as a dancer I had to adjust my under—standing of movement from the ballroom to the bedroom.

BEDROOM DANCE MOVES

Don't mind the pole in the photos; it was just a convenient prop to help demonstrate the very important Hip Drop motion. This motion alone will improve anybody's sexual performance immediately. Remember, the Hip Drop is the motion of the ocean!

HIP DROP (NAIL IT TO THE WALL)

IT'S IMPORTANT FOR guys to get this move down instead of the outdated, overrated "pump" fiction move portrayed in porn. This is where we get to unleash the Lumbar Love Lock's best benefit. I call this version of the Hip Drop "Nail It to the Wall" because that is the easiest way to describe and teach people the most important movement in lovemaking. Here's why: The G-Spot is up and in behind the pubic bone, and the head of the penis has a ridge. To make use of that ridge while in the vagina, the stimulation power is actually more in the pullback than in the push in. Because the Hip Drop emphasizes the pullback, it is very effective at stimulating the G-Spot.

1. Lean your back against a wall with your knees bent, your feet slightly more than shoulders' width apart.
2. Place your shoulders firmly against the wall.
3. Press your palms into the wall for support.
4. Engage your lower abs, curling and lifting your hips forward and up, and repeatedly and rhythmically drop your hips back down, without arching your back, as if using your sacrum (tailbone) to drive a nail into the wall behind you.
5. Practice dropping your sacrum against the wall on the beat to a rhythmic count of four. Then try emphasizing every other beat: hard on one, easy on two, hard on three, easy on four, and so on. Remember to always maintain a forward pelvic tilt, coming to a neutral hip placement when you push back against the wall. Continue until you become fatigued.

NOTE: *This drop-back motion is a much more efficient movement for making love than the pump and push in. Even though it appears similar, it feels very different to both partners. It is especially useful if you want to work the AFE and PFE cervix points, as you will surely see.*

Activity does not mean productivity. Being able to find and then rhythmically and repeatedly press the pleasure points within a woman is essential for both partners' efficacy. Learning to move well allows you both to discover new pleasure points, sometimes because one opens up another.

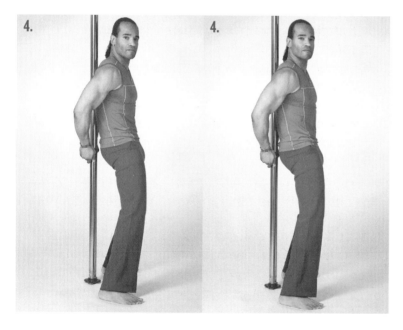

HIP DROP (BALL ON THE WALL)

MICHAEL JACKSON MADE a whole career out of this movement. The resistance you meet by pressing the ball in this exercise will give you power in your pullback by developing your back muscles for that all-important lovemaking backbeat rhythm! Try practicing to "Billie Jean."

1. Lean with your back against a wall with your knees bent, your feet slightly more than shoulders' width apart.
2. Place a soft, pliable kickball at your sacrum, just below the small of your back.
3. Press your palms into the wall for support.
4. Place your shoulders firmly against the wall.
5. Begin rhythmically pressing the ball into the wall.
6. Practice dropping the small of your back against the ball on the beat to a count of four. Then try emphasizing every other beat: hard on one, easy on two, hard on three, easy on four, and so on.
7. Remember to always maintain a forward pelvic tilt, coming to a neutral hip placement only when you push back against the ball.

Once you've mastered this version, try the backward version (not pictured):

1. Stand facing a wall with your arms up, elbows against the wall, your knees slightly bent, your feet slightly more than shoulders' width apart.
2. Place a small kickball against the wall at your pubic bone.

3. Using your pubic bone, press the ball until you feel a strong tension pushing back against you.

4. Begin practicing your press in, and release in a Hip Drop. Continue until you get tired.

CAUTION: *Women need to be careful with this move, as clitoral arousal is possible!*

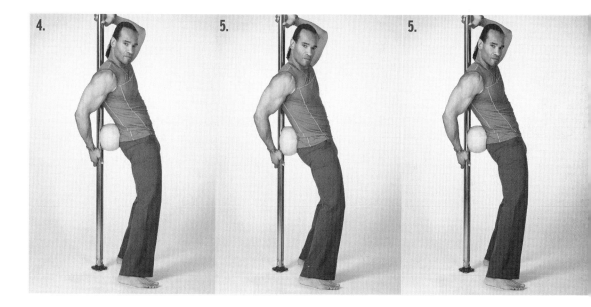

FORWARD SCOOP (COME-HITHER HIPS)

ONE MOVEMENT THAT gets no end of attention is what I call the Forward Scoop, or Come-hither Hips. It follows the shape of a fishing hook, and it's easy to get hooked into it: forward and under, up and pull back. This requires both the Lumbar Love Lock and the Thoracic Love Lock: You push with the Lumbar, then pull with the Thoracic, a combustible combination.

1. Stand with your feet a little more than shoulders' width apart.
2. Relax the lower abdominals and let your pelvic bone drop down. Be sure you do not contract the lumbar muscles to arch the back.
3. Move your hips slightly forward, curling your lower abs upward as if moving your pubic bone toward the ceiling.
4. Pull back, using your middle back muscles.
5. Repeat.

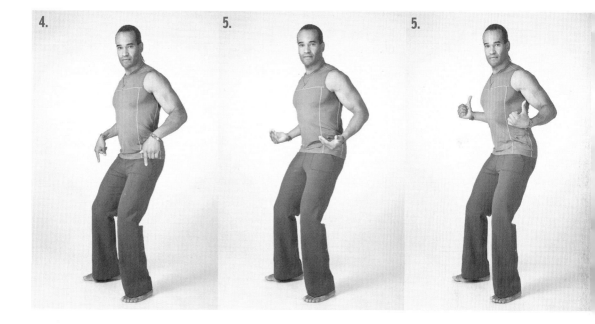

The Forward Scoop's curling-up movement of the lower abs will help the woman to expose her G-spot and the man to access and apply pressure and depth of stroke.

BACKWARD SCOOP

THIS MOVE WORKS better for women, but it is good for men to master as well, as there are certain cueing motions where the man can use it (chapter 5). As in playing pool, cueing is establishing a pivot or contact point from which you can move fluidly forward, backward, up, or down and rotate from side to side to establish accuracy. This helps a couple to more consistently and effectively press on the mutually agreed-upon internal pleasure points. (More on cueing later!) With the Backward Scoop you are backing your way into the Lumbar Love Lock.

1. Begin standing with your feet a little more than shoulders' width apart, your knees slightly bent. Engage a slight pelvic tilt.
2. Engage the lower back, then slightly contract the middle back and spinal muscles so as to bring the hips up and back.
3. Contract your lower abs, dropping your hips down. You should feel your lumbar release.
4. Slide your hips forward to a slight pelvic tilt.

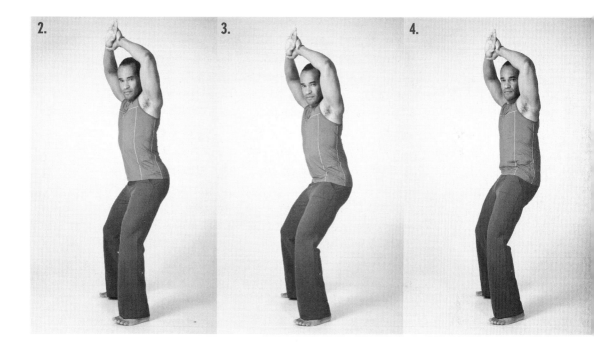

DEEP PRESS

LISTEN UP, GUYS, sometimes it's not how you move, but how you don't. There are times when you can move a woman more by *not* moving than by moving. Sex Magic 101: Just pressing and holding on a spot within her can send her out of her mind. If she says hold still, *hold still.*

Practicing the Deep Press movement builds muscles in the lower abdomen and flexibility in the lower back that will get and hold her attention. You'll find that the Rock the Plank exercise shows its value here, bringing you and your partner to a deeper union. The Deep Press is perhaps the best expression of the Lumbar Love Lock. It's a full-on pelvic tilt to fully press her inner pleasure points. A dual Lumbar Love Lock in a Deep Press on a woman's AFE or PFE is an energy exchange that would overload a Vulcan Mind Meld.

1. Stand with your knees bent, your feet a little more than shoulders' width apart. Engage a pelvic tilt.
2. Contract your middle abs as you engage a much more pronounced pelvic tilt, lifting your pubic bone up and in. Hold it for a count of thirty.
3. Release and repeat. Now breathe through it and try to hold it for a count of forty, and so on.

NOTE: *Remember, you want to practice pulling your pubic bone toward your navel. What you're learning is to practice holding the press position. A woman, at times, just needs to feel that deep physical connection—to feel that the man is present. This is the tantalizing taunt of the press, breathing into one another where no movement moves both of you. The Deep Press also allows your pubic bones to press, potentially stimulating her clitoris. This will often result in a very powerful orgasm for her. Sometimes less is more!*

Dr. Helen Fisher, anthropologist and author of *Why Him? Why Her?: Finding Real Love by Understanding Your Personality Type*, says that the area in the brain stimulated by love, the ventral tagmental, is the same area that registers cocaine. Love is an addiction.

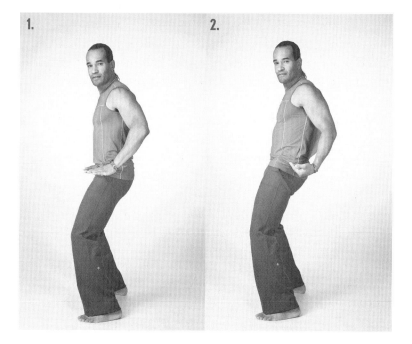

1.

2.

DEEP DRAG

THE DEEP PRESS + the Forward Scoop = the Deep Drag! The purpose of this motion, a strong come-hither hip movement, is to sustain stimulation as you maintain pressure on a pleasure point. The power here is in the pullback; you are simultaneously pressing and holding up while pulling back. A shallow Deep Drag can stimulate the G-spot. A deeper Deep Drag can stimulate the AFE. Practice this move as often as you can—if you master it, you will flatten your abs and raise the roof! A Deep Drag is a great way to leverage your Lumbar Love Lock.

1. Stand with your knees bent, your feet a little more than shoulders' width apart. Engage a pelvic tilt.
2. Inhale. As you exhale, contract your middle, then lower abs, lifting your pubic bone up and forward and holding this pose.
3. As you hold it up and in, slide backward (but not too far back) using your middle back muscles. You want to maintain contact with the stimulation point.
4. Notice the hip height in Step 3 above is higher than in Step 1. This is because you are dragging against the upper inside wall.
5. Repeat in sets of ten.

Remember: A woman's deeper internal stimulation points, unlike the clitoris, respond better to pressure and pressing motions than to friction.

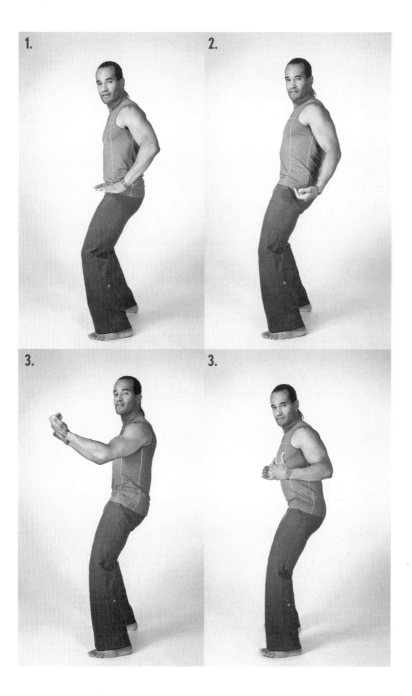

FORWARD-OVER SCOOP

THIS MOVE WORKS better for women, but again, it's good for both sexes to master as the man can use it in certain cueing motions (page 192). We use the pole in the photos just for the fun of it.

1. Stand with your feet a little more than shoulders' width apart, your knees slightly bent. Engage a slight pelvic tilt.
2. Increase your pelvic tilt by deeply contracting your lower ab muscles. Your glutes will also tighten.
3. Slightly contract your middle abdominals, moving your hips forward (lower abs contracted).
4. Release your lower abs, dropping your hips down.
5. Slide your hips backward to a neutral flat-back position.

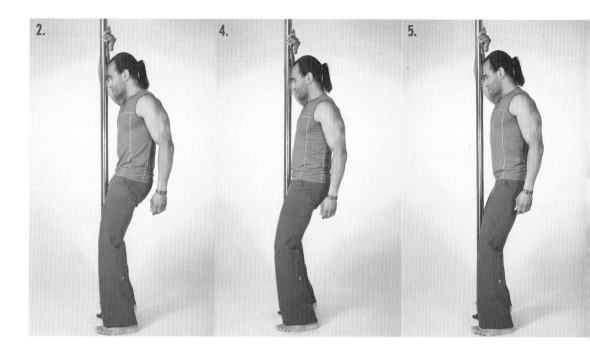

BURLESQUE KICK

THIS AEROBIC EXERCISE will lift far more than your spirits. No ifs ands ors, this will give you a great butt, nice horseshoes (triceps), and hamstrings, too!

1. Sit leaning back on your hands. Do not lock your elbows.
2. Bend your left leg up, resting your sole on the floor with your heel just below your left knee.
3. Engage a pelvic tilt, holding your core muscles tight.
4. As you exhale, prop yourself up into a table position, extending your right leg out straight with your toes pointed, and hold. Your body is now up (semi-flat), your core tight, and your hands and left foot still flat on the floor.
5. Inhale, bend your elbows, and sink your hips toward the floor. Bring your right foot down and place it flat on the floor next to your left. Your glutes should reach a low point without actually going to the floor.
6. As you exhale, begin extending your left foot out straight. As you do, lift your hips up so that your left foot and hip arrive in the up position at the same time.
7. Repeat switching sides at a steady count, one and two and three and four and (left) kick and (right) kick and (left) kick, and so on.

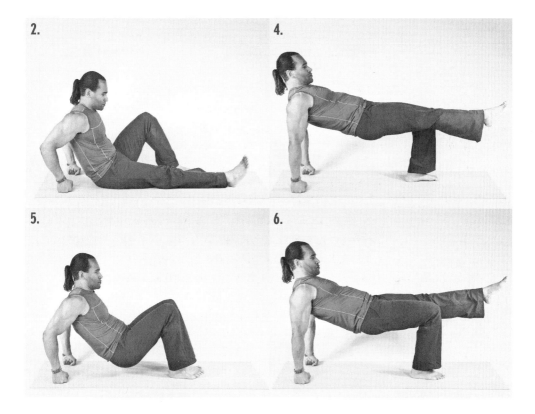

THE SLOW SWIVEL

THIS SLOW SWIVEL involves moving the sacrum in a swivel from below the navel, which is usually the rooting point of your movements. This movement is in and out, from left to right or right to left. Because a woman's internal stimulation points vary, she needs to direct and guide her partner toward those points. In the bedroom, this determines the direction of the swivel. The male pubic bone, which is always somewhat directed upward by the lower abs, determines the pressure. For instance, if her stimulation point is up and to the right, then his swivel must move in from the left to stimulate it. See the section on cueing (page 192) for a better understanding of this process.

1. Stand with your feet shoulders' width apart. Engage a pelvic tilt without moving your ribs.
2. Lift your left hip toward your left rib by contracting your left oblique.
3. Engage your middle abdominals to move your hips forward.
4. Lift your pubic bone up.
5. Lift your right hip toward your right rib by contracting your right oblique.
6. Lower your hip back to a neutral pelvic tilt, keeping your back flat.
7. Repeat with your right hip.

The Slow Swivel is not only internally effective but also externally suggestive—a sexy move that can take people over the edge just by witnessing it. When you practice this one, think of a slow blues or reggae grind and use some music to suit your mood.

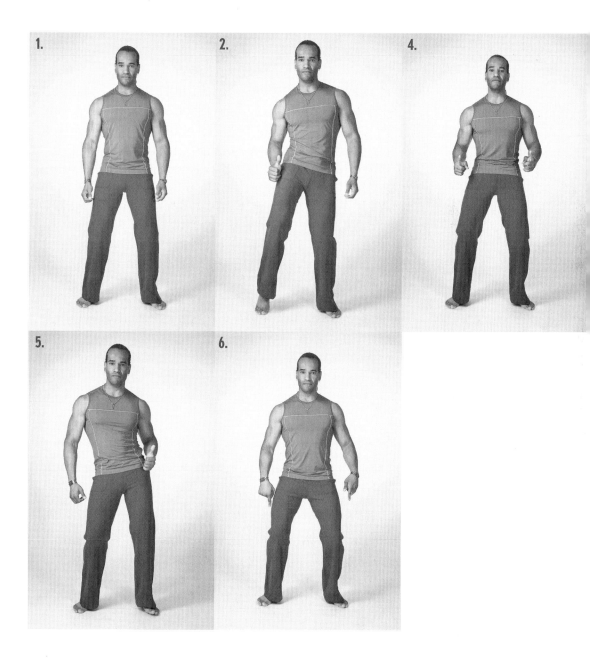

THE SEATED SACRAL SWIVEL (CHAIR DANCE)

THIS IS A variation of the Standing Swivel that you can practice anywhere there is a chair. Be discreet if you can; otherwise you might attract unwanted attention! The Seated Sacral Swivel involves moving the sacrum in a swivel from below the navel, which is usually the rooting point of your movements. This movement is up and in, down and out, from left to right or right to left.

1. Sitting in a chair, bring your feet to a little more than shoulders' width apart.
2. Practice the side oblique lateral lift to one side.
3. Engage your lower abs to create a pronounced pelvic tilt.
4. Try to lift the other side.
5. Return to semi-neutral pelvic tilt, but not a complete release.
6. Rhythmically repeat steps 2, 3, and 4.
7. Try going in the opposite direction.

WHEN I WAS in Japan, I heard a story of a great archer, a *sensei* (master), who was once asked by a Westerner if he could hit a bull's-eye in the dark from a hundred yards away. "Hai," the master replied ("yes"). The Westerner asked, "Can you do it for me here and now?" "Hai," the master said. So a minute or so went by, and the Westerner asked the interpreter, "Why hasn't he shot it yet?" The interpreter turned back to the man and replied, "He is waiting for you to tell him which part of the bull's-eye you want him to hit—upper left or right, lower left or right, or dead center!" That is what I'm talking about when I say you need passion and precision in your movements.

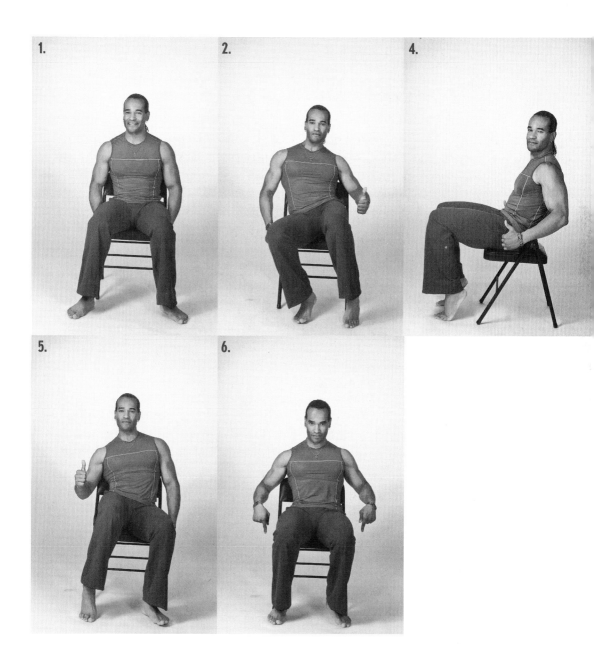

REVOLVERS (BELLY-DANCE MOVES)

THESE MOVES ARE called Revolvers because they revolve in semicircles around the spinal axis. You'll see how the Twist of Fate stretches helped create the flexibility necessary to do these moves well. Revolvers work to increase and improve horizontal hip mobility by engaging your transverse abdominus. I learned these movements from a girlfriend who was a belly dancer, but don't worry, guys; if you aren't into belly dancing, try the Martial Arts Horizontal Movements (below) for the same results!

These moves are especially effective in the Spoon sex position (chapter 5) because learning to rock on your hip bone gives you better articulation than a thoracic thrusting motion. Gentlemen, don't be a Jackhammer Joe!

1. Stand and placing the toe of your left foot forward. Engage a pelvic tilt. Lift your ribs away from your hips. Keep your shoulders and hips square.
2. Slowly bend your right knee, sinking down as if to sit your right hip over your right heel. Stop when you feel the muscles of your right leg and glutes engage to support your weight.
3. Move your left hip forward and over until you can see the outside of your left hip in front of you, or the outer seam of your pants.
4. Bring your hip back so it is even with your shoulders. Maintain your pelvic tilt and your weight steady over the bent right knee.
5. Repeat until your right leg gets tired, and then switch legs.

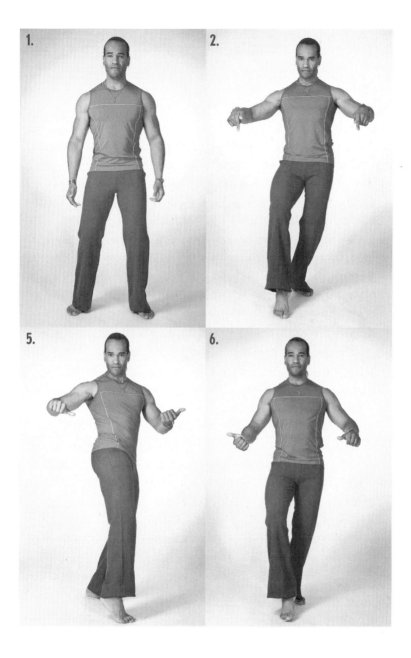

MARTIAL ARTS REVOLVER WITH A KICK

BOYS, THIS WILL help you achieve the motion without having to feel you were belly dancing.

1. Stand and place the toe of your left foot forward. Engage a pelvic tilt. Lift your ribs up and away from your hips. Keep your shoulders and hips square.
2. Slowly bend your right knee, sinking down as if to sit your right hip over your right heel. Stop when you feel the muscles of your right leg and glutes engage to support your weight.
3. Move your left hip forward and over until you can see the outside of your left hip in front of you, or the outer seam of your pants.
4. Lift your left leg, with your knee slightly bent and the sole of your foot pointed inward.
5. Inhale. As you exhale, engage your transverse abs and lower oblique, turn your hip over, and extend a low hooking kick.
6. Inhale and retract your leg back to the Step 4 position.
7. As you exhale, again engage your transverse abs and lower oblique, turn your hip over, and extend a low hooking kick.
8. Continue until fatigued on that side, then try the same on the other side.

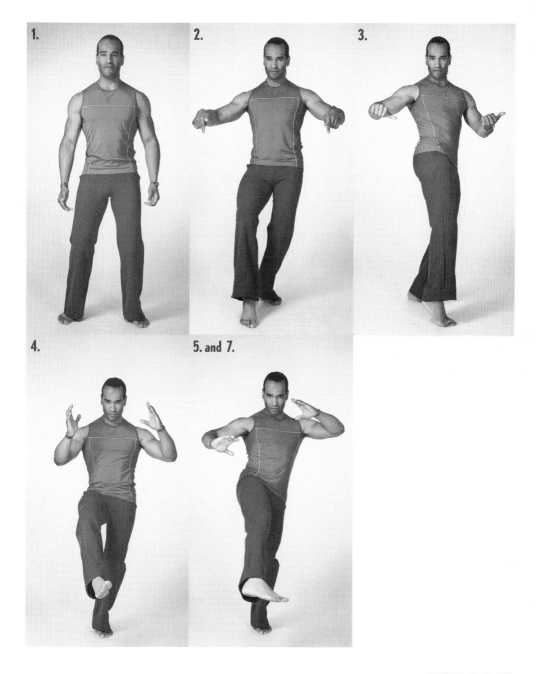

STANDING REVERSE REVOLVER

THESE MOVES WORK to increase and improve horizontal hip mobility. Here, again, you want to engage your transverse abdominus. Like the Hip Drop, the Reverse Revolver gives you the power of the pullback (because of the shape of the head of the penis).

1. Stand and place the toe of your left foot forward. Engage a pelvic tilt. Lift your ribs away from your hips. Keep your shoulders and hips square.
2. Slowly bend your right knee, sinking down as if to sit your right hip over your right heel. Stop when you feel the muscles of your right leg and glutes engage to support your weight.
3. Move your left hip forward and over until you can see the outside of your left hip in front of you, or the outer seam of your pants.
4. Lift your left leg, with your knee slightly bent and the sole of your foot pointed inward.
5. With power, snap your hip back so it is even with your shoulders. Maintain your pelvic tilt and your weight steady over the bent right knee.
6. Repeat steps 2 and 3 until your right leg gets tired, and then switch legs.

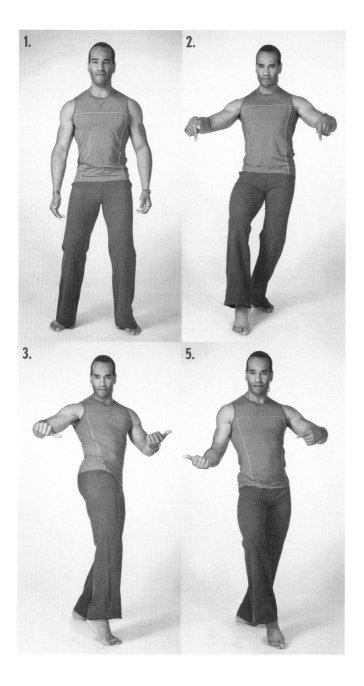

1.

2.

3.

5.

MAYA (SIDE SCOOP OVER)

THIS MOVEMENT WILL cause sensual tremors in the depths of your being that will register on the Richter scale. Get ready for a sexquake! It's called a Maya because it looks like an optical illusion, and in Sanskrit, *maya* means "illusion" in the broadest sense of the word. In the West, it is thought that opposites such as good and evil and yin and yang are separate, whereas in the East they are considered complementary: They blend and depend on each other, as do women and men. It is our perception that is the illusion. Practicing the Maya will give both of you the agility and accuracy to probe and passionately press the pleasure points to greatly increase your lovemaking skills. It also provides a long-lasting visual that will leave your partner shaking their head—or just plain shaking.

1. Stand with your feet a little more than shoulders' width apart, your knees slightly bent. Engage a slight pelvic tilt.
2. Engage and contract your left oblique, lifting your left hip toward your left rib as you drop your right hip down.
3. Contract your left rib, sliding your whole hip to the left.
4. Begin relaxing your left oblique and rib, and contract your right oblique as you drop your left hip down.
5. Slide your hip back to the right to a neutral position.
6. Practice this several times on each side before switching.

My students often describe the Maya as "whittling away the waistline." Dr. Mehmet Oz has said that it is more important to pay attention to your waist than your overall weight.

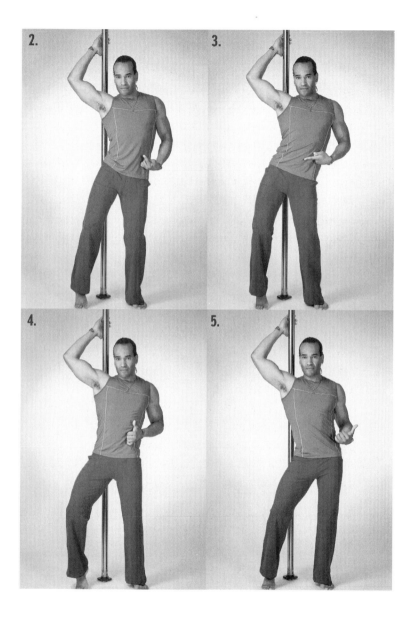

REVERSE MAYA (SIDE SCOOP UNDER)

THIS IS MORE of a lateral scooping movement that looks like you're shovelin' some lovin'. It's similar to the Come Hither Hips movement except that you slide it to the side. Once you add these moves to your practice, you will elevate your erotic status no matter what your previous state. You will sizzle by default.

1. Create a pelvic tilt by contracting your lower abdominal muscles.
2. Drop the left iliac crest (hip bone) down.
3. Slide your hip over to the left, and lift it up toward your rib.
4. Slide your hip back across to the right and return to the starting position.
5. Repeat on the other side.

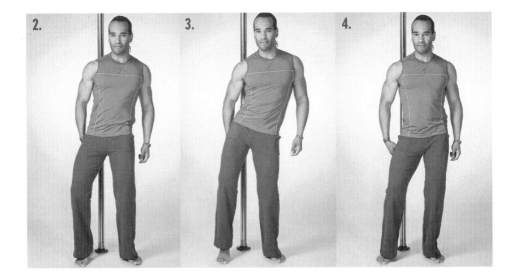

THE PENDULUM

ON OLD MERCEDES cars, the windshield wiper used to swing back and forth from the top. Practice this move and you'll be a luxury lover. Try to do this without involving your legs much. Follow up with the Naughty Kneeling Ninja (page 170).

1. Stand with your knees bent and your feet shoulders' width apart. Engage a pelvic tilt.
2. Without moving your ribs, using your glutes and obliques only, try to move your hips back and forth in a pendulum motion, like an upside-down windshield wiper. You should feel your glutes engage.

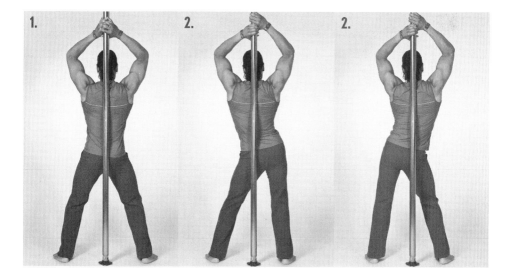

THE POWER IN THE PULLBACK

Sex is like fishing: It's important to set the hook. In sex, this means using the ridge of the penis to rub the G-spot, because the shape of the penis creates more friction on the pullback than on the push. If you move a little beyond the G-spot first, a tight pullback motion while maintaining pressure on the G-spot pleasure point is very pleasing for both woman and man. In figure 21, notice the ridge of the penis and the angle of entry.

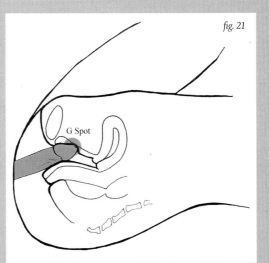

fig. 21

G Spot

MARTIAL ARTS MOVEMENTS

For all those guys who think that dance is for sissies, remember that Bruce Lee, before he made any movies, was the cha-cha champion of Hong Kong. Dancing with a partner and fighting an opponent in kung fu both require attention, skill, timing, and rhythm. As it turns out, *wu shu* is the term most used for martial arts in China, while *wu dao* is the term for dance—and both terms describe the development of kung fu in their respective areas. So whether in the ballroom or the bedroom, vertical or horizontal, learning to move your body well and do it in rhythm is important.

TANTRIC TRAINING FOR the Weight Room: Ask anybody why they rush through their training moves in the gym, and they'll tell you they are trying to get it over with as fast as possible to avoid pain. This is a sure recipe for a lousy lover. Anybody rushing to release "out of pain" while training will rush to release into pleasure during sex. This is very un-Tantric; the Chinese say people do everything in their lives the same way. A rush to release doesn't allow time for an orgasm to mature, or, at times, for the female orgasm to happen at all. It is also why people don't get the results they seek in the gym: If muscle is not allowed to break down because people don't stick around long enough, it can't build up. Am I saying that suffering makes you sexier? Yes, if you do it wisely and willingly!

KUNG-FU FLOOR KICK

THIS ONE WILL test you. Although it features the glutes and triceps, this is a full-body exercise for everyone that will lead to full-body orgasms for sure. These motions will help you adjust to the different angles you have to work with to create or maintain contact and pressure on stimulation points. They also develop power in the hips and glutes for sustained lovemaking.

1. Sit, lean back on your hands, and lift your hips to create a bridge or table with your body. Do not lock your elbows.
2. Bend your left leg up, resting your sole on the floor, with your heel just beside your left knee.
3. Engage a pelvic tilt and hold your core muscles tight.
4. As you exhale, prop yourself up into a table position. Extend your right leg out straight with your foot pointed and hold.
5. Inhale, bend your elbows, and sink your hips toward the floor. Keep your right leg out straight with your foot pointed, and hold. Your body is now up (semi-flat), your core tight, and your hands and left foot still flat on the floor.
6. Exhale and prop yourself up into a table position, extending your right leg out straight.
7. Repeat on one side until fatigued.
8. To switch sides, inhale, bend your elbows, and sink your hips toward the floor, bringing your right foot down and placing it flat on the floor next to your left. Your glutes should reach a low point without actually going to the floor.
9. As you exhale, begin extending your left foot out straight. As you do, lift your hips up so that your pointed left foot and hip arrive in the up position at the same time.

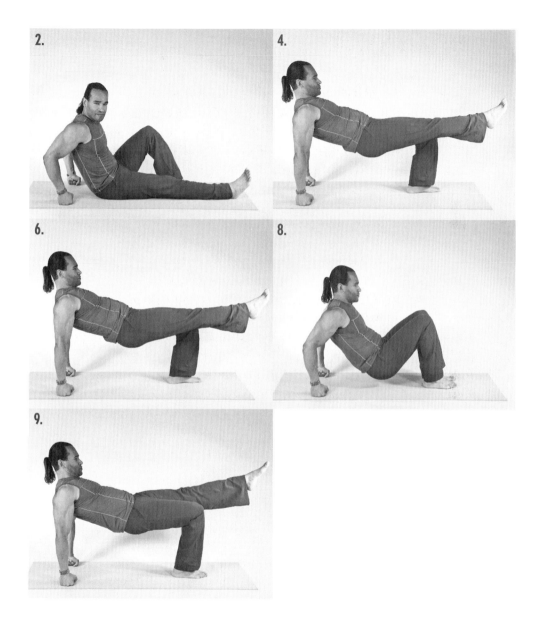

KNEELING KUNG- FU KICKBACK

FOR WOMEN, THIS reverses the effects of gravity on the backside. And guys, women like a little something to grab on to just like we do! Both of the kung-fu kickbacks get their energy from the expansion and contraction of the glute muscles only. It's as if your femur (thigh bone) is rotating like the hand of a clock from your hip.

1. Kneel on the floor on all fours.
2. Engage a pelvic tilt. Keep your core tight and your lower back (lumbar) flat.
3. Lift your right leg up so your knee is at hip height, with your shin and foot pointed straight back. Your shin should look like it is resting flat on a pane of glass.
4. Inhale. As you exhale, slowly extend your right leg (your foot flexed or pointed) straight back to semi-full extension, still as if on a pane of glass. Do not lock your knee.
5. Bring your knee toward, then away from your chest. Try to do this without moving your pelvis.

DR. DANIEL AMEN, a renowned neuroscientist, says, "Men who have more sex live longer. Women who want more sex live longer." During sex, our bodies release positive hormones such as dopamine, serotonin, oxytocin, norepinephrine, vasopressin, testosterone, and human growth hormone—all of which help us to live longer by strengthening our immune systems. Other studies show that the more attractive you find your lover, the more likely you are to powerfully orgasm, releasing even more positive hormones into your system.

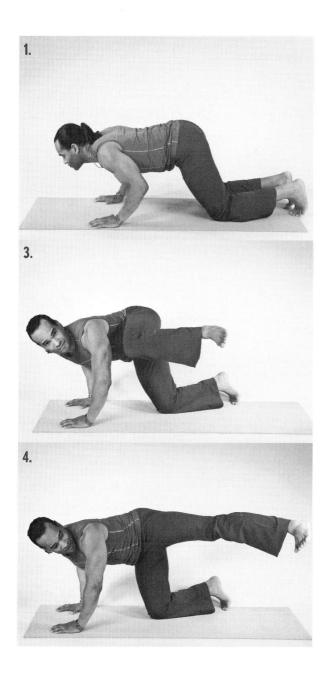

STANDING KUNG-FU KICKBACK

1. Stand on a slightly bent left leg.
2. Bend your right knee and lift it up to hip height, with your leg parallel to the floor. If you need to, place your hands on a support (a chair or countertop). Your shin should look like it is resting flat on a pane of glass.
3. Inhale. As you exhale, slowly extend your right leg (your foot flexed or pointed) straight back to semi-full extension, still as if on a pane of glass. Do not lock your knee.
4. Inhale and bring your knee toward, then away from your chest.
5. Exhale and extend again, trying to lift your foot a little higher. Try to do this without moving your pelvis itself.

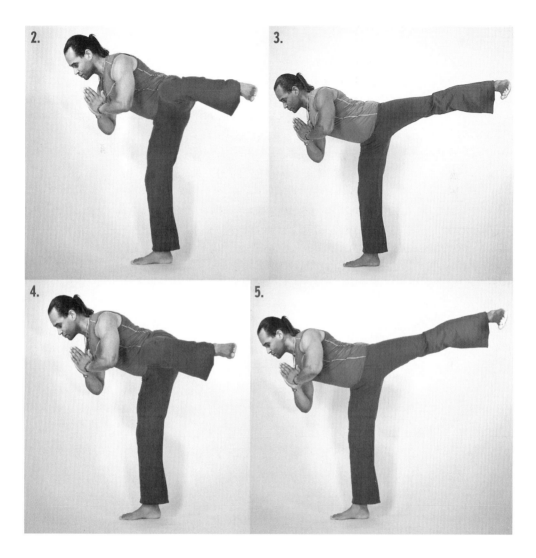

NAUGHTY KNEELING NINJA

LATIN DANCE MOVES that emphasize the use of leg and rib movements (versus the hip and spine focus of our work) may look sexy, but they do not translate to the bedroom! Just to prove to you how small a part your legs actually play in your lovemaking, try this out.

1. Kneel on the floor with your knees a little bit apart.
2. Engage a pelvic tilt and lift your ribs slightly.
3. Try the Pendulum movement.
4. Try the Hip Drop.
5. Try the Slow Swivel movement.
6. Now try the Deep Drag and Deep Press.
7. Pick and choose from the rest of the exercises and try them from your knees.

Notice how little your feet and legs are involved in making love, compared with your hips, glutes, lower abs, and back muscles.

WHEN I WAS a college freshman, my girlfriend slept with my best friend because she thought I didn't find her attractive. The truth was that I was unschooled in any form of the intimate arts. Translation: I was a virgin, and since I didn't know what to do, I did nothing. She unfortunately took this to mean that I didn't want or desire her. My friend raved about how beautiful she was—as did I, but the difference was that he told her and acted on it. Lesson learned: Women need to know that they are desirable to the object of their desire.

NAUGHTY KNEELING NINJA HIP DROP

THE NAUGHTY NINJA Hip Drop from the knees is one movement that every man should learn to do well—a default lovemaking motion. When it's time to get down and dirty and all else fails, "Drop it like it's hot!"

1. Kneel on the floor with your knees slightly apart.
2. Engage a pelvic tilt and lift your ribs slightly.
3. Relax your middle abs.
4. Fully engage your lower abs and create an exaggerated pelvic tilt.
5. Begin dropping your hips (exhaling) and again raising them (inhaling). Maintain a slight forward pelvic tilt, coming to a neutral hip position.

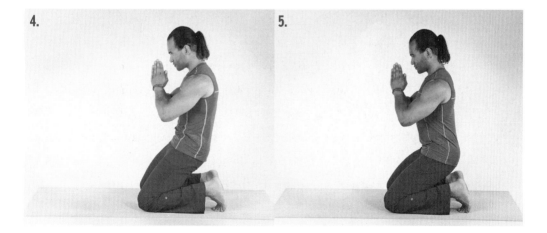

NAUGHTY KNEELING NINJA DEEP PRESS

REMEMBER THAT THE purpose of mastering the Deep Press is to maintain contact with the internal stimulation points that respond best to pressure.

1. Kneel on the floor with your knees slightly apart.
2. Engage a pelvic tilt and lift your ribs slightly.
3. Relax your middle abs.
4. Inhale. As you exhale, engage your middle abs and contract your deep lower abs and glutes.
5. Holding this pronounced pelvic tilt, lift your pubic bone up, in, and forward, and hold it for a count of thirty.
6. Inhale, and release to a neutral pelvic tilt.
7. Repeat step 4, and this time hold it for a count of thirty.

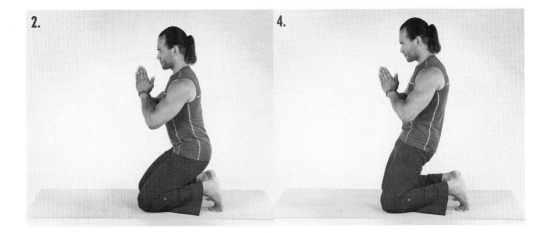

Feathering and Butterfly Kissing: I know, it doesn't sound like the most masculine thing a man can do, but if having her come again and again and again does, consider looking—or should I say licking—into these techniques. There are two times when they are effective: One is when she is on her way up to climaxing, and the other is after she has had an orgasm and either her clitoris or her G-spot is slightly chafed or hypersensitive. Using your tongue (for gentle butterfly kisses on the clitoris) and/or your finger (for feathering, a light touch in a flickering motion on the G-spot) will rearouse her. Once she is rearoused, you can stimulate her more vigorously. Always pay attention to her responses—subtle hints abound.

NAUGHTY KNEELING NINJA DEEP DRAG

THE NAUGHTY KNEELING Ninja Deep Drag is the same as the Naughty Kneeling Ninja Deep Press except that now you will also slide back as you press up. This drag practice, like a strip routine, should be sloooow, deep, and strong.

1. Kneel on the floor with your knees slightly apart.
2. Engage a pelvic tilt and lift your ribs slightly.
3. Drop your pubic bone.
4. Move your hips forward, lift your pubic bone up, and hold it.
5. As you hold it up and in, slide backward (but not too far back) using your middle back muscles. You should feel your glutes engage.
6. Repeat in sets of ten until fatigued.

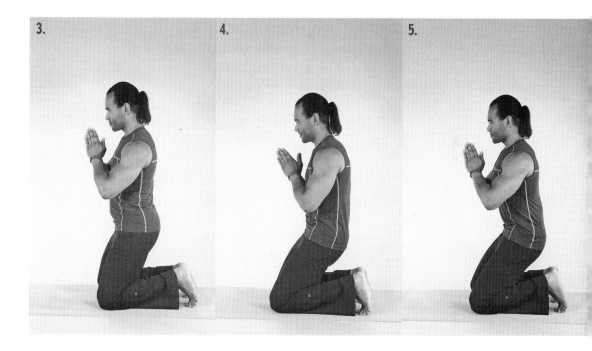

NAUGHTY KNEELING NINJA SCOOP

THE CURLING-UP MOTION of all the lower-ab movements will assist the woman to position herself for the man to access her G-spot, and for the man to access and apply pressure and depth of stroke.

1. Kneel on the floor with your knees slightly apart.
2. Engage a pelvic tilt and lift your ribs slightly.
3. Relax your middle abs.
4. Move your body slightly forward, contract your middle back muscles somewhat, and let your pelvic bone drop down. You do not need to contract your lumbar muscles to arch your back. Rather, your hips should drop down and back because you are relaxing the lower ab muscles.
5. Curl your lower abs upward, as if lifting your pubic bone toward your navel center as in the "Full Tilt" Love Lock.
6. Release your glutes and drop back to the starting position.

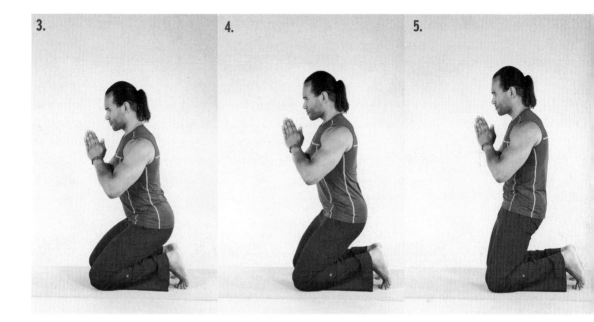

KUNG-FU FLOOR KICK (SIDE SHIFTS FOR OBLIQUES AND TRANSVERSE ABS)

THESE MOTIONS WILL help you adjust to the different angles you have to work with to create or maintain contact and pressure on stimulation points. They also develop power in the hips and glutes for sustained lovemaking. This is different from the regular floor kick because you are executing a horizontal hip shift turn, which works your transverse abs each time you kick. This move will help you do the Spoon position better by strengthening your triceps, glutes, and hamstrings.

1. Sit propped up on your hands or fists. Do not lock your elbows.
2. Bend your left leg up, resting your sole on the floor, with your heel just below your left knee.
3. Engage a pelvic tilt and hold core muscles tight.
4. Inhale. As you exhale, prop yourself up into a table position and extend your left leg out, turning your hip and flexing your foot inward. Your body is now up (semi-flat), your core tight, and your hands and left foot still flat on the floor.
5. Inhale. Bending your elbows, sink your hips down toward (but not to) the floor, bringing your left foot down and placing it flat on the floor next to your right. Your glutes should reach a low point without actually going to the floor.
6. Inhale. As you exhale, prop yourself up into a table position and extend your left leg out, turning your hip and flexing your foot inward.
7. Repeating on one side until fatigued, and then switch sides.

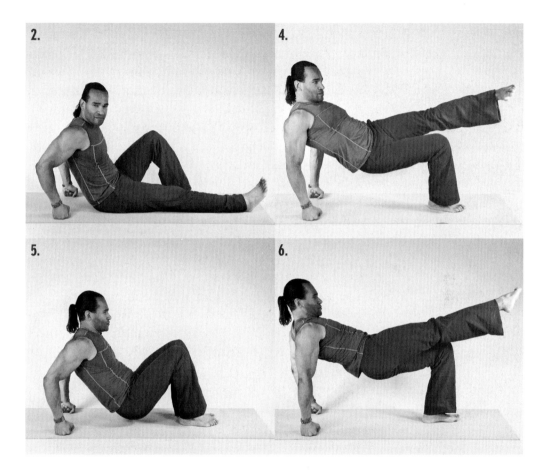

NAUGHTY KNEELING NINJA PENDULUM

THIS WILL PROVIDE the sexy side-to-side motion that will allow you to be on cue for any pleasure pocket she might have.

1. Kneel on the floor with your knees slightly apart.
2. Engage a pelvic tilt and lift your ribs slightly.
3. Without moving your ribs, using only your glutes and obliques, try to move your hips back and forth in a pendulum motion like a an upside-down windshield wiper. You should feel your glutes engage.

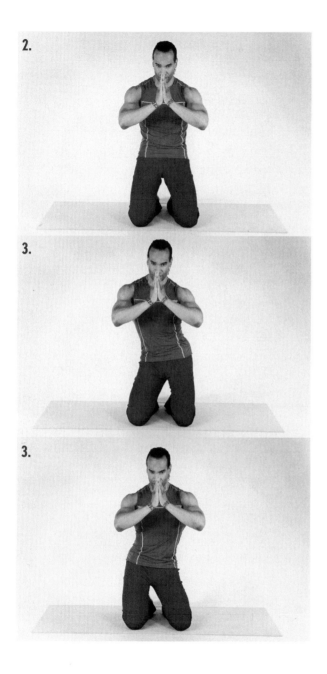

2.

3.

3.

NAUGHTY KNEELING NINJA SLOW SWIVEL

THE SLOW SWIVEL immediately makes any sex position better. Not only does it feel great to your lover, it looks great, too, provided they can see you employing it!

1. Kneel on the floor with your knees slightly apart.
2. Engage a pelvic tilt and lift your ribs slightly.
3. Lift your left hip toward your left rib by contracting your left oblique.
4. Engage your middle abdominals, lift your pubic bone, and move your hips forward.
5. Lift your right hip toward your right rib by contracting your right oblique.
6. Lower your hip back to a neutral pelvic tilt (your back flat). You should feel your glutes engage.
7. Repeat on the opposite side.

The Slow Swivel is an erotic exchange that leaves lovers deranged! The Naughty Kneeling Ninja will help you to execute this killer move.

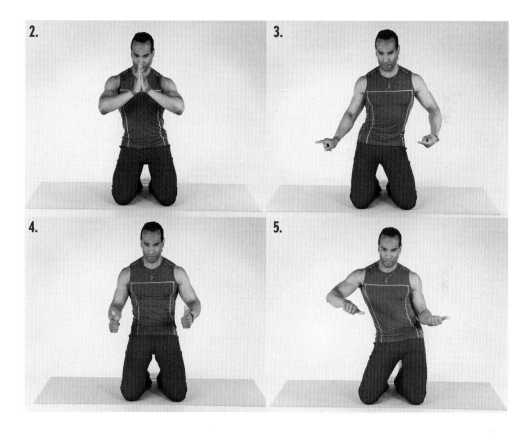

NAUGHTY KNEELING NINJA SIDE SCOOP

THIS MOVE IS like a half dose of the Slow Swivel, but extremely effective at isolating a woman's internal stimulation point.

1. Kneel on the floor with your knees slightly apart.
2. Engage a pelvic tilt and lift your ribs slightly.
3. Relax your middle abs.
4. Relax your lower abs and let your pelvic bone drop down. Do not contract the lumbar muscles to arch your back.
5. Drop your right hip.
6. Slide your hips over to the right.
7. Lift your right hip back up.
8. Slide your hips back over to the left.
9. Repeat ten times, then switch to the other side.

During an orgasm, libidinal energy is released into your system through inner pleasure points that can only be reached consistently with precise, passionate pelvic movements synchronized by two committed partners who have taken the time to learn and understand each other.

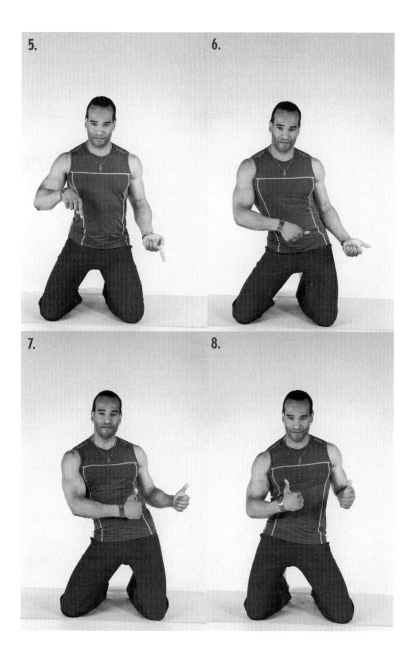

5.

6.

7.

8.

FLYING SIDE BLADE KICK

THEY SAY LOVEMAKING isn't an exact science, but this movement will allow you to move with surgical precision in tight areas.

1. Lie on your left side on the floor, your legs extended, hands flat on the floor in front and back of your body.
2. Bend your left leg, cupping the inside of your right knee with the instep of your left foot.
3. Engage your core muscles so that your lumbar is flat.
4. Extend your right leg, either flexing or pointing your right foot.
5. Inhale and lower your right foot, rocking on the left hip. Feel your right oblique stretch at the lower waist.
6. Exhale and raise your right leg by contracting your right lower oblique.
7. Inhale and lower your leg back down.
8. Repeat until fatigued.
9. Switch to your other side.

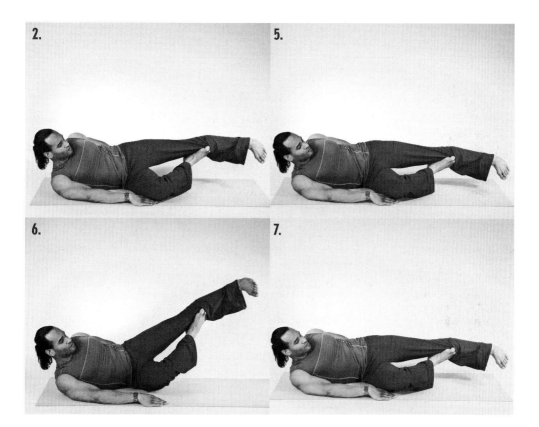

2.

5.

6.

7.

In *Batman Begins*, Henri Ducard (Liam Neeson) corrects his student Bruce Wayne (Christian Bale) when he forfeits his firm footing for a perceived killer strike (in our context, a killer stroke). If you give up rooting, in life and in lovemaking, you can neither live nor make love effectively. You may change how and where you are rooted, but always re-root yourself when you move. It will allow you to be more powerful and precise in expressing your passion.

FROM THE MAT TO THE MATTRESS

5

*m*EN, JUST BECAUSE you've got the (blue) pill doesn't mean you've got the skill. Having more hard-ons doesn't make you a better lover any more than having more golf clubs makes you Tiger Woods—and in any case, you can see where that got him! Unfortunately, there is a pervasive misconception in both the gym and the bedroom that activity means productivity. The quantity of your workout time and sex time may increase, but if the quality doesn't increase and you can't see improvements in the mirror or on her face, you'll end up unhappy. And remember,

"If mama ain't happy, ain't nobody happy!" In both the gym and the bedroom there is grunting, groaning, sweating, screaming, and so on, but people in both settings are constantly sacrificing the quality of movement for the quantity of movement. Many work harder and faster but not better or smarter. (In fact, the reason they have to work harder and faster is that they aren't working better or smarter). In the gym, often to show off, men and women alike use almost twice as much weight as they need to, sacrificing their productivity, development, and inner peace by stressing and straining.

Do you put your heart and soul into working out? What about making out? The top three complaints I always hear from women about their men during sex are:

1. Slow doooown.
2. That's not it.
3. That's it—you stop, you die! (Often when men find the spot, they don't last long enough to get a woman to climax because they come too soon for her to let go completely.)

People make these mistakes in the gym as well as the bedroom: They stop just when the exercise is starting to work, even if they're not doing it in an optimal way. They stop just as the muscle is ready to succumb. The muscular "failure," or seizure, or burning is like the muscle having an orgasm (and people make some of the same faces, right?). Effective exercise and satisfying sex work almost the same way. For exercise, you need resistance, intensity, and duration. For sex, you need pressure, intensity, and duration. In both situations, people have to learn to stay in one place—the right place—long enough for something to happen. The problem is that most people have some form of amorous ADHD. In real estate, exercise, *and* sex, it's about location, location, location.

I believe people spend too much time trying to be sexy and not enough time actually getting better at sex. We all need to become what we want to attract. Sex appeal is just that, the peel—the outside housing of the juice. So are you ready to get juicy? Are you ready to find out how good great sex can really be? Now that you've learned some new ways to move, it's time to get down to business in bed. Whether you want to try a new position or just add spice to the ones you already love, this chapter will give new meaning to the phase "apply what you've learned"! We don't stop playing because we get old; we get old because we stop playing. So lighten up and laugh a little while you're lovin'.

According to experts on *Oprah* (yes, I watch *Oprah*), 40 percent of marriages are sexless, 70 percent of women fake orgasm, and 40 percent of married women have never had an orgasm. Sadly, some men think this is women's fault. One woman on the show had been married more than twenty years and had kids, but had never had an orgasm. Her husband had the nerve to say, "It's not my fault. I know what I'm doing." Does that seem fair? Guys, if you're an electrician and the lights don't work in your house, guess whose fault it is?

HOW TO MAKE ORDINARY SEX POSITIONS EXTRAORDINARY

You don't have to become a "sexpert," acrobatic contortionist, or Tantric master to have great sex. You can enrich your love life by applying these simple techniques to whatever position you'd like! Remember, it's not the position that's important; it's how you and your lover move together in those positions that matters.

TURN ON A DIME   Take a dime and put it on a table in front of you. Pick up a pen and circle the outside of the dime with the tip of the pen, moving from your elbow. As you are circling the dime, notice the range of motion in your wrist. That is about as much motion as you need to make love well (well, give or take an inch). How do we know this? The female G-spot is about the size of a dime, sometimes a quarter. Now move the pen forward and backward across the dime. Notice again how much movement is actually involved. Remember, a woman's inner stimulation points are literally a bundle of nerves, and respond better to consistent pressure than intermittent pounding. I know, pounding looks good, but would you rather have it look good or work?

I once heard a Cuban drummer saying that the mambo bars in Cuba don't have enough room to move, so people dancing have to express all their soul and passion in about one square foot. Two people in about a square-foot space moving tightly and in sync—sound familiar?

CUEING   Have you ever played pool? If you look at the way the pool cue is used, there is a pivotal point, an axis created by the hand resting on the table that maneuvers the point at the end of the cue stick. The point where the hand rests on the table corresponds to

The ins and outs of intercourse are about how to stay *on* the spot so you get *off* more quickly. Once a couple has successfully started stimulating a point, if the woman moves back two inches and her partner moves back two inches they have collectively moved back four inches and are off the spot they want to stimulate. Sex is about micro movements that produce macro results, so pay very close attention to the art of staying very close.

the point where a man's lingam meets a woman's labia, her vulva, and pubic bone. Friction there, at the clitoris, in the right position is important, but for our purposes now we will address how a man's "cueing up" can affect the inner sanctums of a woman. In pool, you will notice that as you move the maneuvering hand to the left, the tip of the cue goes right; if you move the maneuvering hand to the right, the tip goes left. The same applies in intercourse. When you move your hips left, the tip of your lingam will move right. If you move your hips down, the tip of your lingam will move up inside her yoni. It's like a seesaw. If you move your hips up and to the right (from your perspective), the tip of your lingam will move down and to the left inside of her.

Swivel pivoting is much like a big gun on a fighting ship. If you move the gun down twenty degrees and to the left thirty degrees, the barrel will aim twenty degrees up and thirty degrees to the right. To see this for yourself, take a

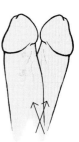

← To move the head right   To move the head left →
   Move your hips left   Move your hips right
fig. 22

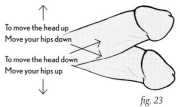

To move the head up
Move your hips down

To move the head down
Move your hips up

fig. 23

pencil or pen and lay it down in front of you. Place one finger on top of the pen in the middle, and try pushing one end to the left. Notice which way the other end moves.

Lingam is the Sanskrit word for penis, and *yoni* is the Sanskrit word for vagina, or, as Oprah calls it, the "va-jay-jay."

MIRRORING The mirroring exercise is a great way to learn to see things from your partner's perspective. If you're facing someone and you hold up your right hand and they hold up their right hand, their right hand will be to your left. If you want to mirror them, you must do the opposite of what they do. When a man moves to his left, mirroring takes place because of cueing. Now it gets interesting: When his hips move left, the tip of his lingam moves to her left within her yoni. If the man moves his hips right, his lingam will move right within her. So if she tells you to move to the left inside her, move to your left (unless you're behind her, in which case, of course, everything is backward: You move right to stimulate her on her left!).

Here are a couple of examples for you. In this picture, I have moved to my left and am holding her right leg, supporting myself with my left arm, to achieve the angle I need for an interior stimulation point to her left. In the next example, she is actually pointing her left leg out to her left to verify that. Here I shift to my right, now holding her left leg, supporting myself with my right arm to stimulate her inside on her right. Here is the same pose with her leg pointing to the right.

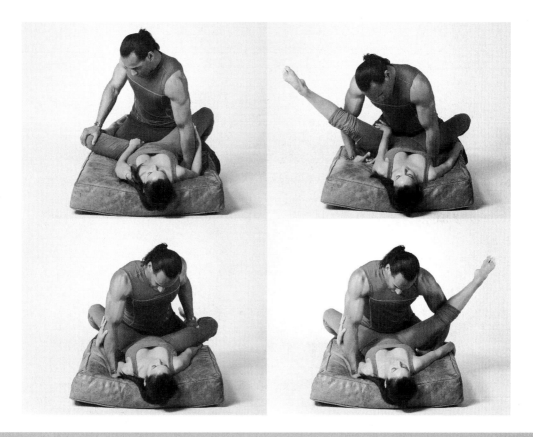

When lovers both move in the same direction, it cancels the movement out completely. Sex, in order to serve both partners' needs, counts on countering. This is why cueing, mirroring, and understanding how to turn on a dime are important physical aspects of turning each other on during intercourse.

CUEING QUIZ

1. To move the head of the penis up, which way do you move your hips?

2. To move the head of the penis left, which way do you move your hips?

3. To move the head of the penis right, which way do you move the hips?

4. To move the head of the penis down, which way do you move the hips?

5. To move the head of the penis up and to the left, which way do you move the hips?

6. To move the head of the penis down and to the right, which way do you move the hips?

ANSWERS:

1. Down

2. Right

3. Left

4. Up

5. Down and to the right

6. Up and to the left

MIRRORING QUIZ

1. If you are behind her and she says move down, you move in which direction?

2. If you are behind her and she says move down and to her left, you move which way?

3. If you are behind her and she says to her right, you move which way?

4. If you are in front of her and she says to her left, you move which way?

ANSWERS:

1. Up

2. Up and to the right

3. To your left

4. To your left

HOW TO USE A BED BETTER

As I mention in Cueing and Mirroring, the angle and position from which a man enters a woman will directly affect what happens for the woman internally. Of course, she is responsible for serving as his guide, a copulation copilot if you will. But sex is not just about angles and positions. It's about how you feel about what is happening. Your sexual position will never be as important as the psychological and emotional position you enter into sex with. Physical entry is only an invitation, not the end but a means. Men, be aware that your partner is opening not just her legs but her world to you, and that when a man enters a woman, she also enters him. At the moment of entry, not just two people but two entire worlds engage one another.

As you begin making love, allow yourself some nonverbal sexual small talk. Don't just go right to work. Introduce yourselves physically as if meeting for the first time. I often recommend holding a position, a press, and a deep, shared breath, really feeling each other first. Acknowledge each other, continuing the eye contact, the touching, and the stroking of each other's bodies. Kiss, kiss, and then kiss some more! Men, play with her hair a little, stroke her face. Ladies, show him you have confidence in him. It can be animalistic, too—you can grab, squeeze, or spank a little if you know that's what your partner likes. As you combine communication and playfulness with some pressure on an inner plexus (of nerves) through mirroring and cueing, sex becomes a simple pleasure.

In the **Missionary Position G-spot** (fig. 21), notice that the entry is an up and in motion, not the typical straightforward thrusting that men sometime use. The Hip Drop works really well here. You can press and hold, but you do not need to press deep. As you can see, the G-spot is not that far in. Remember, short strokes lead to long orgasms!

So tell me: How could there be a sexual revolution when there was never a sexual evolution? The only concerns during the sexual revolution were more sex and birth control—not better sex. They were about the right to have sex, not the need to have it right. Is there a right way and a wrong way? Maybe not, but there are ways to make sex much more satisfying for both partners.

With the **Missionary Position AFE** (fig. 24), his short stroke is a little deeper, but it's short nonetheless. Here a Deep Press is sure to impress. Again, go up and in, but more in than up. Always remember: In missionary position, lifting her legs up and back (sometimes accomplished by putting a pillow beneath her hips) not only exposes the G-spot but also shortens her vaginal canal. Men who might consider themselves challenged in the length of their "third leg" must learn to shorten the distance they need to run!

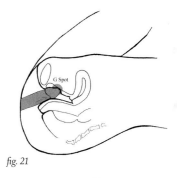

fig. 21

USUALLY AFTER AN orgasm there is reveling, cuddling, and caressing. Occasionally there is something different—crying and laughing. Should this occur, do not panic. On a rare and most beautiful occasion, a woman can have a profound orgasmic experience that will bring her to tears. She may have experienced an emotional upheaval, and you have but one job

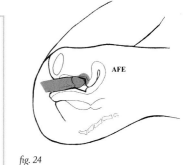

fig. 24

at that moment: Hold her! Be with her! Stroke her hair! Rub her cheek! Support her! Tell her it's okay to let it all out, and that you are there for her. She may then start talking about what she experienced, and man, if there's ever a time in your life when you need to pay attention, to listen, this is it. You are about to hear something that has deeply affected her, and you don't want to miss or misunderstand it. It may be something that greatly helps you understand her, and maybe understand yourself.

The **Missionary Position PFE** (fig. 25) shows how to stimulate the PFE at the back of the lower vaginal canal. Notice the down and inward positioning of the head of the penis. The man wants to press and rub the PFE passionately until it allows her a release. Remember again, these points respond best to pressure, not pounding, so his movement should stay close and tight.

In the **Doggy Style G-spot** (fig. 26), if he is going to stimulate this area from behind, he needs to get very much down and in, as the G-spot is in and down behind the pubic bone. Think of trying to spoon the last bit of jam from the jar; the results will be sweet for sure.

With the **Doggy Style AFE** (fig. 27), keep in mind again that she'll be down and out if he doesn't go down and in. Again, this is where cueing comes in: To go down and in, the man moves up for a downward stroke. This is a good position to practice his pressing prowess on her AFE.

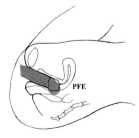

fig. 25

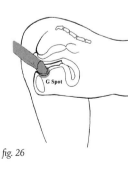

fig. 26

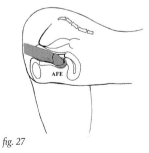

fig. 27

The **Doggy Style PFE** (fig. 28) shows that there is an up side to getting down. What was once down is now up, and of course in. Remember the song "Ring My Bell"? That's what is happening here: It's just like ringing a doorbell. The man must keep pressing on the button until he gets an answer!

The **Pin-down and Pin-up Doll G-Spot** (fig. 29) are good opportunities for some cueing tips. Tip 1: The angle of approach is downhill, so the man must maneuver his hips up to get down. He must lie on her back and use short, sweet strokes. The angle of approach for the Pin-down Doll and the Pin-up Doll have a lot in common. Tip 2: In the Pin-up position, as she will be leaning slightly forward, his line must be straighter because of her simulated downward slope. This allows the man a wonderful opportunity to do some neck nibbling while he's slow-stroking.

Is it time for **Pin-down Doll AFE** (fig. 30)? Is she lying on her stomach smiling over her shoulder again? Never keep a woman waiting! Remember the Rock the Plank movement? This is where Daddy needs to be a deep diver. A Deep Press here will release untold treasures of the deep. Cueing Tip 3: Think Kamikaze dive-bombing.

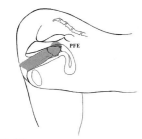

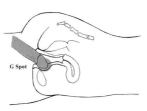

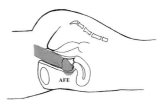

fig. 28

fig. 29

fig. 30

YAB YUM STRADDLE

TRY USING THIS as a meditation position. Sit together, with the woman straddling the man as shown in the photo. Breathe each other's breath: She breathes out as he breathes in, and vice versa. From this position it doesn't appear that the man can manufacture much movement, but the operative word is *appear*. The truth is that the man can lift the woman slightly, providing a saddle by placing his arms under her legs and derrière. He can then assist by supporting her weight and helping her to maneuver, guiding her hips toward and away, forward and back, providing a powerfully passionate and precise penetrative movement. You can also both practice a simultaneous Hip Drop; as the man employs the Hip Drop, she can engage her horizontal Swivel to increase mutual pleasure. Build those biceps, boys, you're gonna need 'em!

The beautiful thing about sacred sexuality is that, more than a union of bodies, it is a union of opposing yet complementary energies that mirror and reflect one another. What makes sex sacred is that it is each individual's quest for wholeness through union with the other. Wholeness is where the word *holy* comes from.

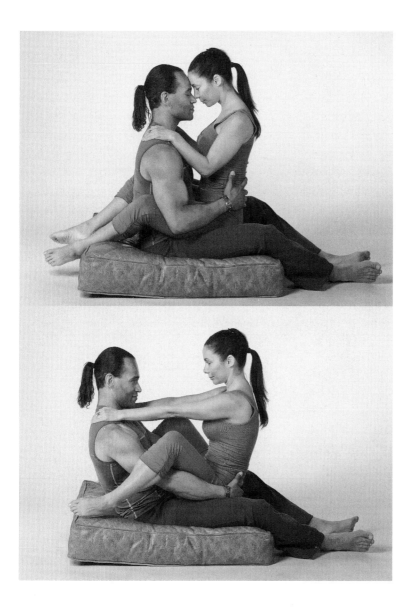

THE SPOON

PERHAPS THE MOST loving position for most of us is the spooning position. I often joke to my male students and friends that when it comes to women, "No spoonin', no forkin'!" But it's really all about the cuddling, and ladies, men love cuddling—no kidding. Cuddling also releases oxytocin, which is often referred to as the bonding hormone.

In the spoon position, because the friction of the sheet restricts you, it is not practical to try to slide back and forth in the traditional push-pull pumping method. The best movement in this position is a Transverse Twist combined with a Hip Drop, pivoting from the side of your hip on the neck of your femur. Remember, men, that you are not pumping but *pressing* and *massaging* the internal stimulation points, such as the G-spot or the AFE and PFE.

It is also nice to lift her top leg up and put your top leg over her bottom leg. This allows you access to her clitoris for manual stimulation. From here, you can Swivel, Hip Drop, or Deep Press for AFE and PFE stimulation while stimulating her clitorally to an earthshaking blended orgasm.

Showing your body is easy. Showing your heart, especially if it's been hurt, is difficult for fear of future injury. As Rumi says, "Love comes with a knife, not some shy request. Half-heartedness doesn't lead to majesty!" Honesty and trust will crown you king and queen of each other's hearts. Hiding what hurts (or, worse, lying) will lead to crowns of thorns.

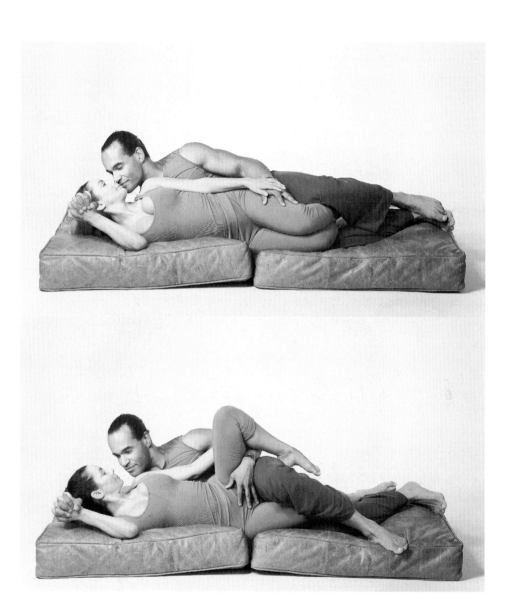

MISSIONARY PRECISION

ALTHOUGH THIS MAY seem to be the simplest, even the most boring of all the sex positions, that is only true if you haven't looked deeper. The missionary position provides a liftoff point for some of the most amazing climaxes possible. Everybody knows about putting a pillow under the woman's hips, and most people know that raising the pubic bone aids in exposing the G-spot. We also know that lifting a woman's legs or pressing her knees back allows a man deeper penetration because it creates a pelvic tilt. A pelvic tilt not only raises the pubic bone, exposing the G-spot, but also, in the process of curving the lumbar spine, releases pelvic tension and shortens the vaginal cavity. When the lumbar is curved by the pelvic tilt, it opens up energy pathways by allowing the spine to relax from the tension normally placed on it by the psoas muscle, which attaches to the lumbar vertebrae from the neck of the femur. This position creates great comfort and, forget ye not, comfort for a woman aids orgasms.

The next thing for the man to remember is to use a passionate, precise Hip Drop motion (as shown) to allow strong and constant stimulation. Try experimenting with the Deep Press and Deep Drag to see what works for her. Always allow the possibility, through pelvic friction, for clitoral stimulation. Just keep in mind that the inner stimulation points respond better to constant pressure rather than to the typical, overemphasized, erratic pumping that causes only intermittent clitoral rubbing. The woman may like to manually stimulate her own clitoris; the man can then back off a little and allow her some finger room. It is also good to add a little lubrication to the clitoris to avoid chapping.

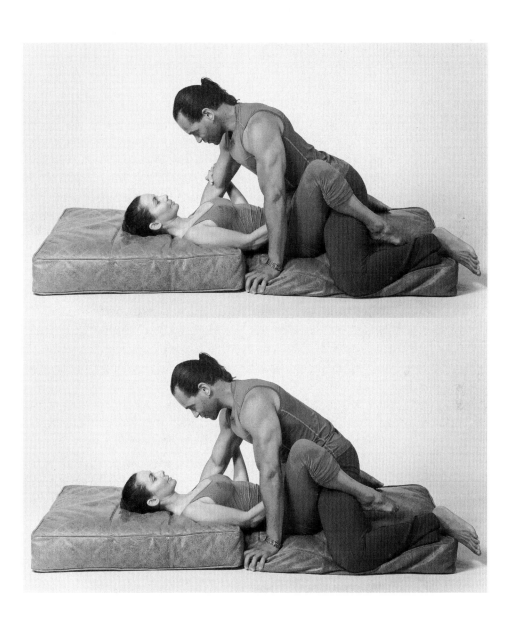

DOGGY STYLE

WHAT WE'RE TRYING to do here is to prevent what is affectionately known as Doggy Style from becoming "dogma" style. This position is often seen as bending over and taking it, which is far from true; the purpose of this, like any other position, is to find a stimulation point. This is a good way to access the AFE, which from this angle is located at the lower rear of the cervix. Since the woman's hips are at around a forty-five-degree angle, her vagina is now shortened. Notice the short, tight hip-drop motion in the pictures: Here I am reaching around to stimulate the clitoris to create the possibility for a blended, if not at least a clitoral, orgasm for her.

Always remember that her stimulation points in this position can be not only down and in, but also left or right.

A VARIATION OF Doggy Style could be called "Froggy Style." If the woman kneels on the bed and sits back between her heels, this comfortably stretches her lower lumbar and opens her hips. If a man enters her from behind in this position, her vaginal canal is greatly shortened and her innermost points (especially her PFE at the base of her cervix) are much easier to access. This is very much an up and in motion for the man, and the woman must be on a chair, couch, or bed so he can position himself below her to enter at an optimal angle. Here, he wants to practice the Hip Drop and/or Deep Press, and hold.

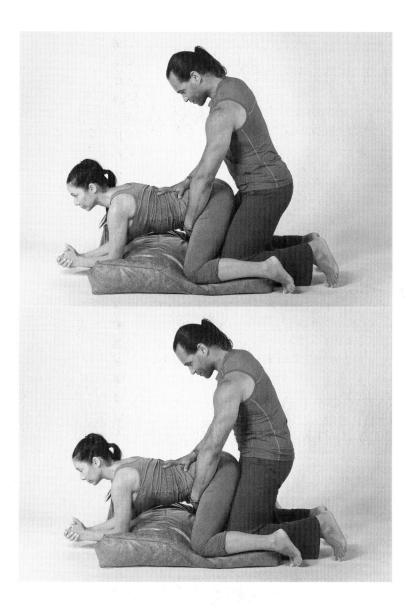

CUTTING CORNERS

THE CORNER OF the bed (or sofa) can be nice because it allows the man to bring his lover literally to the edge, and move in a lot closer to her with his legs posted on either side of the corner. This works well whether she is facing him or not. If she is facing him, she can straddle him and he can support her almost like a modified Yab Yum. She can also lie back with her sacrum propped up with pillows, providing a better angle for G-spot stimulation. Or she can lie comfortably facedown, straddling the corner with one or both legs up and around him (as in A Leg Up, page 222), resting for a relaxed rear entry. Here again, the man can also stand behind her, reaching around to manually stimulate her clitoris if desired. He should try the Swivel, Hip Drop, or Deep Press for PFE stimulation to create a beautiful blended orgasm.

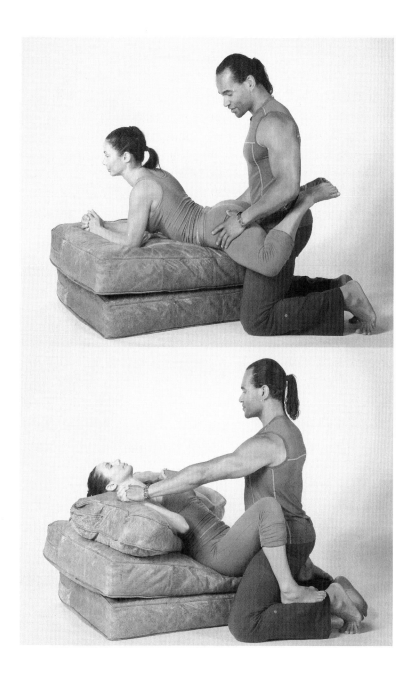

THE SADDLE

THIS IS A variation of the Yab Yum Straddle, a kind of corralled cowgirl! Here the man lifts and supports the woman with his forearms and hands caressing her buttocks, supporting most, if not all, of her weight. In this way she can relax and ride without much energy or effort. With her legs up, her vaginal canal is again shortened to allow greater access to her cervical hot spots. A short, tight Hip Drop motion by both partners, more up and down here, can easily stimulate her G-spot. It also works great if the man lies back, giving him an even better angle to work with her G-spot.

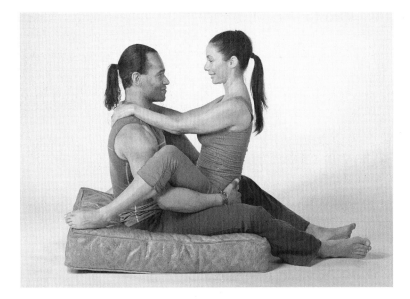

Erotic enabling is the enemy of intimacy. Not being real about how you feel and what you need is lying to your lover. These little lies can be the cause of big pain for both partners. Faking orgasms is ultimately the denial of a beautiful experience and opportunity for both partners to grow, so be real and talk to each other!

THE SLED

THIS IS A variation of the Yab Yum Straddle. Here, the man lifts and supports the woman with his forearms and hands caressing her buttocks, supporting most, if not all, of her weight. In this way she can relax and ride without much energy or effort. She is chauffeured in a slide and glide to climax from any chosen internal point. With her legs up, her vaginal canal is again shortened to allow greater access to her cervical hot spots. It also works great if the man lies back, giving him an even better angle to work with her G-Spot.

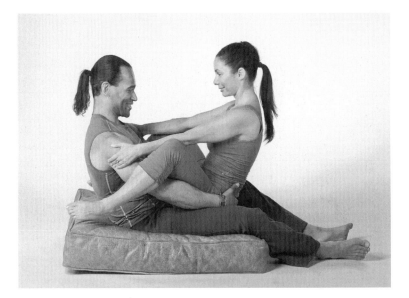

THE EDGE-OF-BED SLED

THE MAN SITS on the edge of the bed with the woman straddling him, but this time his feet are on the floor for leverage. He can put his arms either under her legs (best) or around her waist to guide her hips towards him. This can also be done on a chair, provided it's a sturdy one.

The Edge-of-Bed Sled looks similar to The Saddle (shown below), but is set up closer to the edge of the bed or couch. In this position, the glide and slide movement is a little more effective for stimulating the AFE and PFE than the G-Spot.

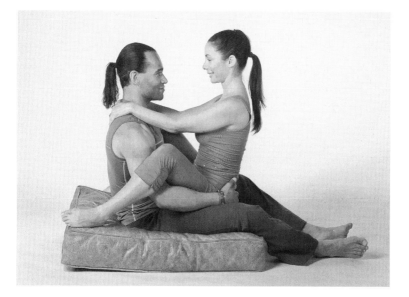

ROCK THE STRADDLE

THIS IS A playful version of the Yab Yum Straddle. She sits with her legs over his, leaning back, holding his hands. The couple can now work with a rocking-chair, seesaw motion to make her G-spot and AFE more easily accessible. Because she is leaning back, her pubic bone is lifted to provide easier G-spot access. She can press down in a Backward Scoop and he can press up in a Deep Press. Guys, you want to Rock the Plank, or rhythmically rock your hips in a Hip Drop motion. Remember where you're aiming, and stay on target.

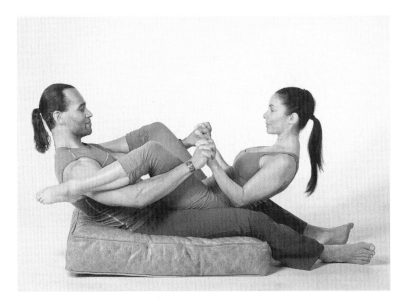

FINDING LOVE IS like finding oil: You can't expect to strike oil if you dig multiple shallow holes.

IN THIS POSITION, the woman is facedown on the bed. The man drops his hips straight down from above hers to enter. He then comes up and adjusts to a motion that's literally straight down and in. The man now has the ability to provide her with an internal massage using Hip Drop, Swivel, Deep Press, or Stop on a Dime! Just remember to maintain constant pressure. He is looking to work on her G-spot in a straight down-and-in motion (see fig. 29, page 201). If he drops back and down a little, he can go deeper and work on her AFE, which will now be on the bottom (see fig. 30, page 201). He can reach around and manually stimulate her G-spot.

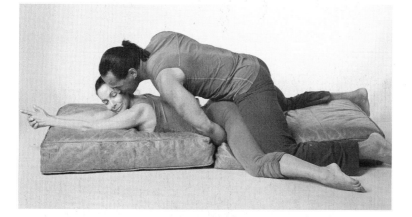

HOW TO SUCCEED ON THE SOFA

A sofa is a bed with a backrest that can offer simultaneous comfort and support for lovers. It is important for the man to occupy a position where his hips are lower than the woman's so that his up-and-in motion can access stimulation points such as the G-spot and the AFE. A down and in motion (Deep Press) will stimulate the PFE area.

UPWARD AND INWARD BOUND

THIS IS A sweet sofa position if the man kneels in front of the woman (the women are liking this already) while she is reclined and relaxed. The main reason this is effective is that he is below her (the women are *really* liking this), which gives him a great angle to stimulate her G-spot. It almost mimics the gyno-chair. This also gives him a perfect, comfortable angle for oral and manual stimulation.

Another juicy position is where she is lavishly draped over and across the back of the couch, facedown, with one leg comfortably (comfort is all-important) over the arm of the couch. (This position is similar to the Pin-up Doll, but leaning over a sofa.) If she is propped up slightly, her G-spot and AFE are more accessible. If she lies down more, her PFE is more open. With her leg lifted at about a ninety-degree angle, she can be entered from the rear, from which position the man can more easily reach around for manual clitoral stimulation. Remember, pleasure point accessibility is always linked to angle change and the woman's pelvic positioning. It is up to both partners to establish comfortable entry and movement positions. She must be able to present herself and receive from a functional angle and position, and he must make sure she is comfortable and he is in a position where he can smoothly enter, access, and stimulate the mutually acknowledged pleasure point.

The female orgasm is God's gift to man. Any man who's ever really given a woman a profound, deep orgasm where she lets go completely, crying out and writhing from the depths of her being, will not deny this. It is something he is compelled to see again and again and will forsake his own orgasm to witness. He will forget about conquering the world. He has borne witness to the divine.

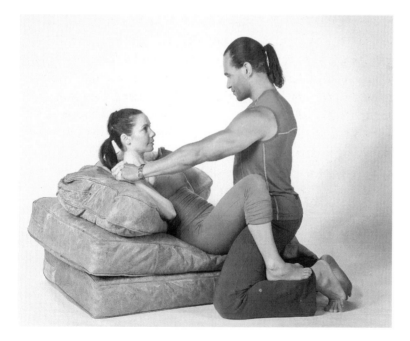

THE COWGIRL STRADDLE

WHEN THE WOMAN straddles the man in this cowgirl position, it is empowering for her, but the need to support her own weight sometimes takes away from her ability to relax. The man can make it easier for her by supporting her, holding her at her waist just above her hips to give her a lift (even to get more downward pull), or even holding hands to support her and establish a nice connection. Try to keep your respective pubic bones in constant contact with each other, as the friction between the two provides clitoral stimulation, which can lead to a blended orgasm.

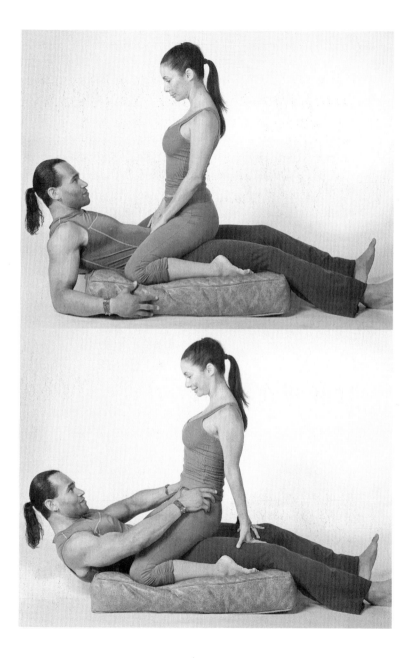

STAND AND DELIVER

A LEG (OR TWO) UP

IN THIS POSITION you have a "leg up" on your way to a sweet climax. The women lies on her stomach on the corner of the bed. Her leg(s) across the top of his hips as he kneels in back of her provide a great pelvic angle that allows not only easy access to her PFE but also wonderful maneuverability and opportunity for closeness and articulation. Which of her legs needs to be lifted depends on which side of her upper vaginal wall her PFE is located. Because you're looking to stimulate deeper points, try the Hip Drop and Slow Swivel, maintaining constant pressure and pressing motions to her deeper points. Remember, there won't be much if any pelvic separation, as you will want to stay close.

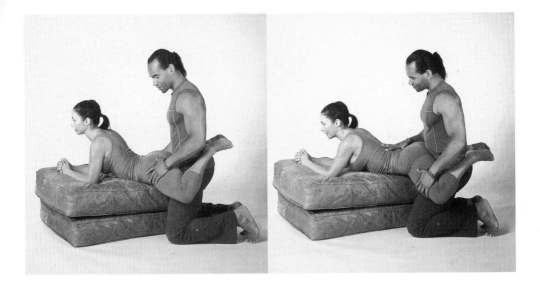

You can also try this on the sofa, where she can pick up a leg and lean on the back of the couch. This is comfortable for her and a good position for the man to provide clitoral stimulation.

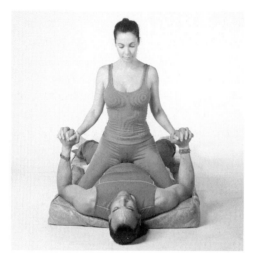

The Leg Up positions all provide great opportunities create a blended orgasm by both stimulating her clitoris and accessing her internal erogenous zones. Her internal hot spots are inner nerve bundles, so have fun playing with these positions and find what works best for you and your partner. You're just nudging nerves and bumping bundles!

STANDING LEG UP

THIS POSITION IS similar to Cutting Corners, but it can be done in various ways. Both partners can stand, with the man standing in front of the woman and holding her leg up; or she can sit across the angled top corner of the couch. Again, the man needs to know which side her stimulation points are on.

WHEN A WOMAN has an orgasm, she moves into a Zen-like state of relaxation. If her fight-or-flight amygdala brain center is firing, or if she has too much cortisol in her system, coming to orgasm is very difficult for her. She must be hot and bothered—aroused—but also cool and relaxed.

THE DANCER

IN THIS POSITION, the man gently pulls the woman's leg up and around his waist, supporting her as he enters. His motion will be a press and rub—short, straight in, and direct for her G-spot. He should use a Deep Press for PFE access at the base of her cervix. For the AFE, which is now on top, he can angle up using a Deep Drag, which is still quite "pressing" but more like a rub, an internal massage of her inner back wall near her spine. Guys, be sure not to arch her lumbar too much as this will decrease her energy flow, which she needs to experience enough stimulation for orgasm.

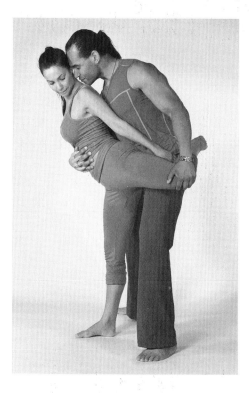

THE SWING (MODIFIED SLED)

YET ANOTHER OPPORTUNITY to make use of the Sled! This time the man is standing, his forearms again forming a sled on which the woman can slide, moving fluidly forward and backward. This works best if her hips are kept close to his. Again, ideally the woman's hips should be slightly higher than the man's to give him better mobility and access to the G-spot and other areas. The man should always keep his knees bent to create a pelvic tilt that will allow easier entry and access to the G-spot, and to avoid back injury. It also helps a lot if her back is against a wall or she can support her upper body. Remember, you want the woman to have little (if any) responsibility for supporting herself.

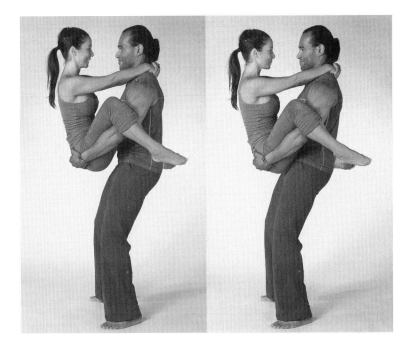

MANY WOMEN HAVE fantasies of being taken. This is not degrading *if it is what she likes!* First, stand her against the wall face in, as if to "stick her up." Then drop down below her to enter, first at an upward motion, then adjusting to more of a straight-in motion. You now have the ability to access her G-spot and AFE zone. Remember, you are Hip Dropping for consistent stimulation on her pleasure points. You can also Swivel, Deep Press, or press and hold, but maintain constant pressure. Think of intercourse as an internal massage. You also can reach around and manually stimulate her clitoris.

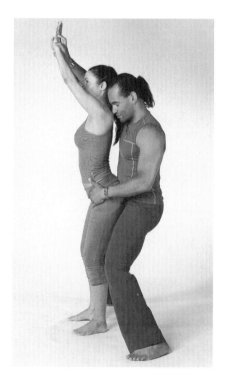

MEN, ALWAYS REMEMBER to keep stimulating her until you notice that she has completely finished with her orgasm. It should be obvious from her breathing and shuddering, but if you can't tell, ask.

THE RHYTHM SECTION:
Tandem Movement

The purpose of the following tandem moves is twofold. Yes, they can help you achieve orgasm, but, more important, they are a way to achieve deeper connection. Learning to truly move together is the ultimate intimate meditation. Most people think of meditation as sitting with your legs crossed in silence among incense and candles. Although candles and incense set a nice mood, what we want is to really feel each other. Whenever you drop into a meditative space it intensifies your focus and awareness of yourself, your partner, and what is happening between the two of you. These moves and grooves are for full immersion, enjoyment, and connection. What you are essentially looking to do is establish a rhythmic movement tandem. You want to drop into a zone where you are both moving in tight precise swirls, strokes, and holds, with the man pressing on the woman's release points. These are precise rubs, where you knead the spots that need it the most.

The "Fit for Love" program is not about how to pick up women. In fact, it's exactly the opposite—it's about how to stay with them!

THE DOUBLE HIP DROP

THE TWO OF you must always find and agree on one spot, one internal stimulation point to work with, be it the G-spot, AFE, or PFE. You then want to sync your simultaneous Hip Drop movements in one steady rhythm together. As soon as the head of the penis reaches the desired internal point, both partners move their contact points slightly away, their hips moving together. When he is returning up from his Hip Drop and heading back up, she is (hip) dropping down onto him. There is only a slight disconnect internally, an ever-so-slight pull away, so that the head of the penis still stays in contact with the desired and agreed-upon inner contact point. (Remember the dime-size movement?)

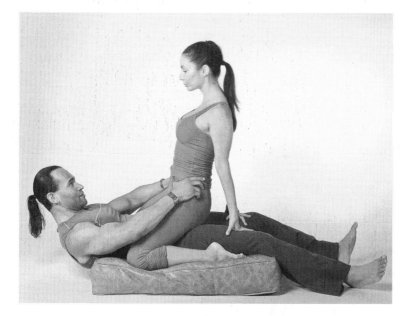

Here are two versions of the Double Hip Drop to try. The starting position for both of these is the woman on top, straddling the man in a seated position. Once you learn to do this consistently, you will be able to transport each other to a new space through timing.

1. As soon as the hips get beyond the opposite way (moving apart), begin moving the hips back together. (If you hear hip skin slapping, yes, it sounds good, but you've gone too far!) Here, the man's penis is inserted semi-deep (an inch or two) behind the woman's pubic bone to persistently press the G-spot while externally providing another pleasant surprise. What's the pleasant surprise? Because of the pelvic proximity, the woman's pubic bone should rub against the man's, allowing simultaneous stimulation of the G-spot and clitoris. Be careful: In this position, there is every possibility you may develop a friction addiction!

2. A deeper version of this move can also give a sweet stimulation at the AFE and PFE, near the cervix. It's the Hip Drop movement done just as you did it for the G-spot, only in a deeper way and place: the cervix. It is still possible during this move to stimulate the clitoris with a relentless rubbing action, allowing the pubic bones and the chosen deep spots to stay in constant contact. Remember, when the woman is on top, or sitting upright, her cervix drops down so it is easier to access. Ladies, remember to avoid the common cowgirl mistake of bouncing up and down, and instead rock the pelvis in your Hip Drop.

THE DOUBLE DEEP PRESS

IN THE DOUBLE Deep Press, both partners agree on a stimulation point to focus on within the woman. When she acknowledges that the pleasure point is being pressed, the two of you press together: The head of the lingam presses up and in, and her pleasure point within the yoni presses down onto the head of the lingam. Together they simultaneously pulse in the Deep Press, barely moving with an ever so slight yet intense rocking motion. It is an internal dance—a torrid internal tango. You constantly apply more or less pressure, but never let off until someone is getting off (or about to), unless you want to prolong the experience. Then, of course, you can either stop in order to build up more energy, or allow whichever partner feels as though they are ready to go over the edge of ecstasy to do so. This is a good maneuver for men, as holding pressure on a stimulation point and *not moving* can often send her over the edge. It is also a wise way for a man to keep from releasing too soon. In other words, it's a win-win situation.

Then, of course, repeat.

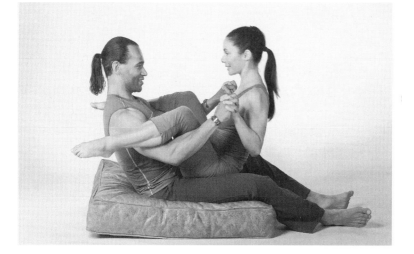

THE DOUBLE DEEP DRAG

THIS HAS A similar starting position to the Double Deep Press. Here the two of you press forward, him up and into her, and she down and onto him. Then hold into each other and slowly and sweetly slide slightly back away from each other, not releasing pressure or pleasure. The idea here is to have you both individually visualize her pushing down and onto him and dragging away, and he pushing up and into her while dragging away. Repeat.

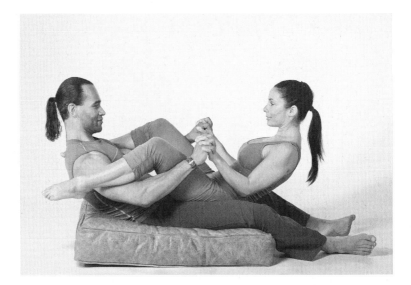

Did you know that both men and women have similar erectile tissue? This tissue is called corpus cavernosum, and it makes up the legs of the clitoris that ride down the outer labia on a woman (fig. 31) and the erectile tissue of the penis on a man. It's no wonder the female clitoris gets erect just like a man's penis. Just as the G-spot and the prostate mirror each other in function, so too do the penis and the clitoris.

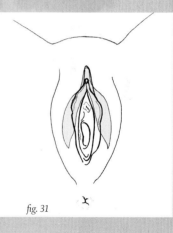

fig. 31

THE MILKSHAKE

HERE YOU SEE her doing a Slow Swivel lifting (opposite you) right, center, and left.

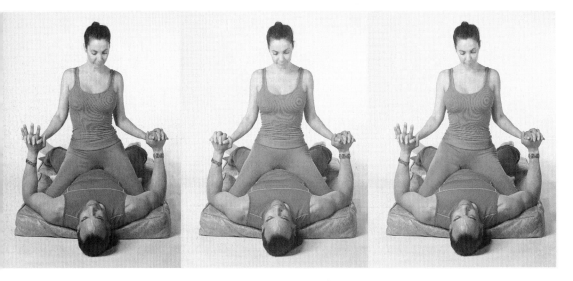

This is truly a climactic tactic. Here, the female is on top, swirling and swiveling as the man Hip Drops her to heaven. Again, because of the close pelvic proximity, clitoral stimulation is an option, and so is the possibility of an extended blended orgasm. This motion provides multidirectional stimulation on a mutually agreed pleasure point. The man, using a Hip Drop, Deep Press, or Deep Drag all together, turns you into an old-fashioned milkshake machine!

You can't really get into sex unless you're into each other, and that is where spirituality comes in. I'm not talking about woo-woo stuff, although I do like candles and incense. I'm talking about sex as a means of mutual expression and exploration as opposed to mutual masturbation.

THE WET TORNADO

THIS IS A simultaneous Slow Swivel, with persistent pressing in on each other while Mirroring each other's left or right movements. This can be done to access the deeper stimulation points or at the G-spot, which is a more shallow penetration.

Ladies, if you are in cowgirl, be sure not to do the typical galloping motion. With its intermittent hopping motion, the typical bouncing up and down of the cowgirl position is not nearly as effective or intense as the rapid ringing of your divine doorbells provided by a tight Hip Drop or Slow Swivel. Wonderfully, these more effective motions allow for the possibility of a blended orgasm because of the relentless clitoral rubbing.

For G-spot stimulation, it works well if she is in a jockey position (cowgirl leaning forward). This allows her knees to move back, causing her hips to create a pelvic tilt. The friction caused by her pubic bone rubbing on his abdomen also allows for clitoral stimulation.

> THE MOST IMPORTANT—and welcome—thing you can do for a woman, other than arousing her, is to relax her. In fact, if she's not relaxed, arousing her alone may not allow her to achieve orgasm. Unless her amygdala (home of her fight-or-flight worry system) turns off, turning her on will do no good.

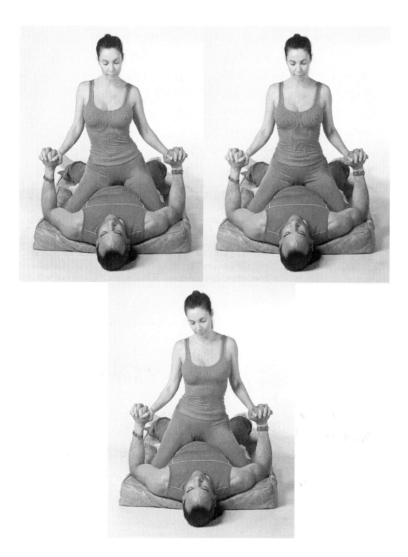

MASSAGE AND MORE

I mentioned earlier that sex is a religious experience, and what would religion be without the richness of ritual? Preparation for a night in together is just as much a ritualistic experience and an honoring of the divine as anything else you will do. After all, you are entering each other's sacred space and temple! Here you have an opportunity to prepare the space with candles, incense, or warming oils as part of a ritual of devotion to one another. And giving each other a sensual massage is a perfect way to start the arousal process and bring eruptive energy flow to the genital areas.

Massage is a combination of exploration and collaboration. The giver may feel somewhat vulnerable, as they are trying both to relax the receiver and to pay attention to what he or she likes. Feedback from both parties is very important, so remember to express appreciation for what you like and give gentle instruction about what you don't like. A good massage will both energize and relax. The following techniques should feel great using nice lotion or massage oil. Does your lover have a favorite scent? Women's sense of smell is stronger than men's, so make sure you find out what scents she likes. Lavender, ylang-ylang, and even baby powder are nice, and licorice can be an aphrodisiac for both women and men.

STARTING POSITION   You want to make your lover comfortable: He or she should lie facedown, head to one side, looking away from their most tense side. Starting at the trapezius muscles (shoulders), work your thumb into the neck and base of the skull, using your four fingers on the front of the trapezius as an anchor. Then press with your palms and knead lavishly with your thumbs. Always ask if the pressure is okay. Turn your hand sideways and massage up and down the neck muscles on the side of their spine, again anchoring four fingers on one side, kneading the other with the thumb. Slow is usually better, although an occasional "quick, quick, slow" pattern is nice, too.

The occiput (base of the skull) and the sacrum (back of the hips) are two localized areas where stress and tension can build up. These areas hold pain, but can also be amazing pleasure pockets when pressed and rubbed the right way. (Ladies, just think about the song "Rub you the Right Way," by Johnny Gill). The occipital and sacral areas are both junction boxes. The occiput is where all the nerves we talked about (with the exception of the vagus nerve) enter the brain stem. The pelvic and pudendal nerve enter the hips through the sacral area, between S2 and S4. The hypogastric nerve enters the pelvic area through the lumbar region. Think of the spine from the occiput to the sacrum (the brain to the booty) as the sex signal superhighway. Obviously we want to take very good care of these Tantric tollbooths!

Begin by slowly pressing and rubbing with both thumbs in a circular outward motion on the lower dot areas (fig. 32). Eventually you want to work your way up the neck to the higher dots. Use light pressure unless you are asked for more. When you reach the

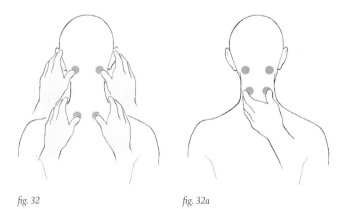

fig. 32   fig. 32a

upper dots at the base of the skull, make your circles more compact. Press up and in, and add a little more pressure as needed. You will feel indents where the muscles connect. Try pressing and holding these spots. Ask for feedback on how it feels.

You can also do this with one hand (fig. 32a), using your thumb and middle or index finger to squeeze and rub while pressing inward toward the spine. You may want to hold your partner's head with your other hand for better leverage.

Now, from these outer dots, massage inward toward the center dot (fig. 32b), continuing to press and rub in a circular motion. Again, try pressing up and in and then hold. This should feel fantastic for the recipient and provide them with immediate relief. You may notice your lover getting vocal around now, but don't stop, as the best is yet to come.

This dot in the center of your occipital area indicates the "Oh!" spot (fig. 33). You want to take your middle finger, or two as shown, for more support, and press up and in. Try small circles as you press. You can support your partner's head with your other hand to increase your "loverage" and dig deep. Press hard and hold until instructed otherwise. Often pressing this spot results in a "braingasm" and is *very* relaxing for the recipient.

fig. 32b   fig. 33

Starting at the small of your partner's back, massage the muscles surrounding the spine. Try pushing the palms of your hands into the spinal muscles (one hand on either side of the spine) and slowly moving up the spine. Add your thumbs and try veering off to the sides of the spinal muscles. Remember, you are trying to clear the pathways for orgasmic energy to rush unencumbered to the brain during orgasm. Feel free to use your palms for overall rubbing of your partner's back muscles and your thumbs for more acute areas that need attention. This is also a good opportunity to read your partner's nonverbal cues. The less dialogue and conversation they have to enter, the better. Think about what feels good when someone is massaging you, and do the same for them.

MOVING DOWN THE SPINE

WHEN I LIVED in Florida, I worked with a machine called the Power Plate, originally designed by the Russian space program to keep astronauts in shape in outer space. The machine used vibration to increase the intensity of whatever exercise you did while standing on it. It was supposed to decrease blood pressure, stress, and cortisol levels and increase serotonin and neurotrophin, leading to a better mood and sense of well-being. It supposedly increased production of the Human Growth Hormone (HGH) as well, thereby increasing metabolism, bone density, and collagen production, resulting in a loss of body fat and a toning and tightening of the skin. I was skeptical at first, but after doing research, I saw many parallels between the Power Plate and Tantric practices, including the massage technique I like to call Spinal Tapping, where partners tap each other's sacrums to stimulate the sacral nerve and the coccyx to release Kundalini.

SACRAL MASSAGE TECHNIQUES

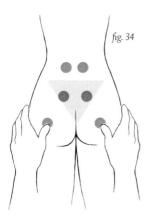

fig. 34

Start in the upper dot area shown at the lumbar and work your way down to the lower dots, using both hands. Working on these points should give great relief to whoever receives it. Remember to press and rub. Try a circular swirl with your thumbs. The middle sacral spots, like the middle occipital point, are legendary for an almost orgasmic release for the receiver. Tap the triangle area of the sacrum, either with the palms of your hands or with grouped fingers (four or five tips together). Massaging, tapping, or causing vibration in this area awakens it and sets up the body for a more profound and intense orgasmic experience through the nerves it serves. Massaging the glutes releases pent-up energy as well.

PELVIC AND PERINEAL massage are like tilling the soil before planting. Massaging the perineal floor, for both men and women, can greatly increase the potency and intensity of orgasms, especially if the muscles have been strengthened by the exercises in this book. Remember, an orgasm is a sexy seizure: It is an implosion of electric energy that can permeate every cell of your body and being.

PELVIC AND PERINEAL MASSAGE

This massage feels extraordinary and can exponentially increase the intensity of orgasms for both men and women. It will also help the uterus, especially during menstrual cramping, as you work toward the middle of the lower abdomen. This also helps loosen up your Sacral/Coccyx Love Lock, allowing you the liberty of full energy flow from the floor of your core. These are very sensitive areas, so it is important to use lubricant, oil, or cream while massaging them, and ask your partner for feedback.

Warming up a woman's stimulation points—allowing them, like the penis, to swell and preheat before intercourse or as part of intercourse—greatly increases the chance of immense, intense pleasure for both partners. It builds the trust essential for taking intimacy to a higher level and can be especially helpful for a woman (or a man) who is having difficulty reaching orgasm. It is unfortunate that many people treat erogenous zones, especially their own, like erroneous zones!

PELVIC/PERINEAL MASSAGE ON A MAN OR WOMAN

1. Have your partner lie on the bed with their knees bent.
2. Kneel in front of or beside your partner.
3. You will be using both thumbs to massage, so place the index and middle fingers above the pubic bone, along the hips.
4. Press and ride both adductors (inner-thigh muscles) with your thumbs, inward from the root in the deep groin and outward toward the knees. (This muscle is shaped like a carrot: thicker at the groin, thinner at the knee.)
5. Massage the perineum muscles with the index and middle fingers of one or both hands, combining presses and circular motions.
6. Massage the glute muscles, especially where the glutes attach to the hips, pressing down and in with your index and middle finger.
7. Continuing the glute massage, try a smooth squeezing motion with your thumbs and fingers, using massage oil, cream, or lubricant.

Orgasm is not an end but a means. It is a beautiful, shared occurrence as part of the ongoing lovemaking act between two people.

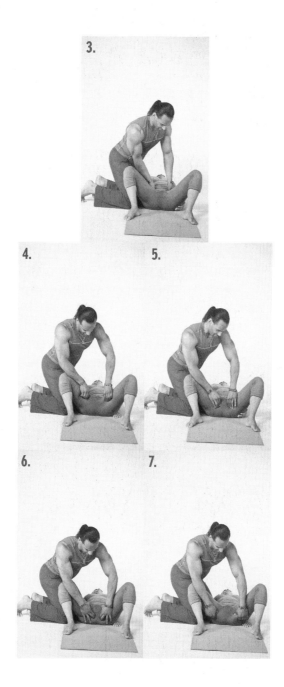

PELVIC/PERINEAL MASSAGE ON A WOMAN

1. Gently introduce your well-lubricated fingers to her vulva and vaginal area.

2. Begin gently rubbing and massaging, sweeping up and down in the soft area between her vagina and anus. (Note: Avoid actually entering the anus.) A gentle semi-pinching and upward stroking of the inner and outer labia as well as rubbing of the vulva is a nice start to the vaginal massage.

3. Notice the crossed arrows on the perineal floor and the thin arrows up and down at the labia, outside the vaginal lips (fig. 35). These are nice areas to stroke, and since most men don't have long fingernails, it is okay to use the index or middle finger to spot-press up and down beside the labia. Using your thumbs to press and rub, try making circles by the arrows beside her vagina. Be gentle in the area just below her vagina. For the longer arrows at the adductor muscles, press or squeeze the muscle gently starting near the genitals, and move outward toward the knees, your thumbs on top, fingers on the bottom.

4. For clitoral massage, make sure she is ready by paying attention to her breathing and, of course, by asking. Using well-lubricated fingers, place your left hand above and on the pubic bone and spread the vulva with two fingers, pulling back with the root of the finger joint to lift the clitoral hood. You can then gently massage her clitoris with the finger of the opposite hand. With the index finger, slowly start with linear, then circular or light flickering motions according to her liking. This should last for several minutes, with reassuring eye contact unless she wants to close her eyes to feel more. If she is aroused to a point where she wishes

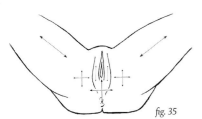

fig. 35

to orgasm, allow her to do so. Maintain the same motion, maybe a bit more vigorously, until she is almost finished. Do not stop until she is finished, but do be aware of when she is done so that you don't irritate her after an orgasm. She will be ready soon enough to be stimulated all over again, or you can, if she likes, gently rearouse her before she completely returns to an unaroused state. You can restimulate the clitoris as a part of this "new" stimulation or move to another stimulation point like the G-spot.

For the G-spot, try slowly and gently inserting your lubricated fingers (fig. 36), usually one at a time until she is ready. The G-spot stimulation is more of a gentle, come-hither motion, pressing up, gently pulling out, and then returning to the original start position slightly past the G-spot. Remember to stay in contact with the G-spot area within her, which feels like the soft-ridged skin at the roof of your mouth.

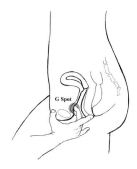

fig. 36

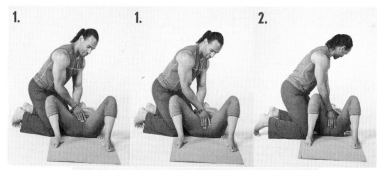

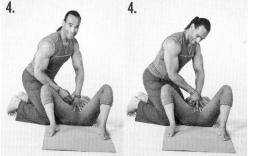

PELVIC/PERINEAL MASSAGE ON A MAN

SINCE A MAN has no vagina, his perineal floor is solid, but we men also greatly enjoy perineal massage. You can use the same pressing-in on the perineal floor as shown in Pelvic/Perineal Massage on a Woman (below, and on page 244). Pressing in the adductor muscles, as well as stroking the area between the anus and scrotum, works well for us guys.

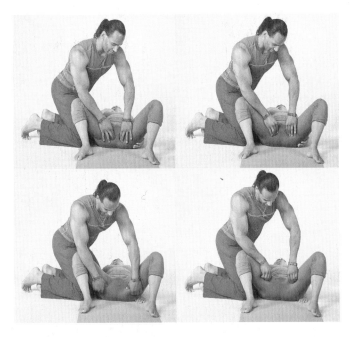

1. Gently introduce your well-lubricated fingers to the area beneath his testes.

2. Begin gently rubbing and massaging with a sweeping up-and-down motion from his anus to his testes, and then gently pressing into the pelvic floor muscles in circular motions.

3. Use the arrows in Figure 37 as a guide. It is probably easiest for you to use your thumbs to press and rub; just be gentle with the middle arrows just below the scrotum. Try to make circles at and around the centers of the arrows as well. For the longer arrows at the adductor muscles, use the semi-viselike grip with your thumbs on top and fingers on the bottom. Press or squeeze the muscle gently, starting near the genitals and moving out toward the knees.

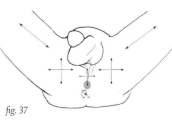

fig. 37

4. His P-spot is opposite your G-spot. You have to enter through the anus. With a well-manicured index finger, you may slowly insert a finger into his anus (fig. 18, page 24).

5. About two inches in, you will find his prostate. A gentle sweeping, pressing, come-hither motion in that area is very soothing and increases overall sexual pleasure. For men not comfortable with anyone entering their anus, you can also stimulate the prostate by pressing upward and inward just in front of the anal opening (fig. 37). You will notice a convenient indent there to access the prostate. A pressing, semi-pumping motion, done gently, will also stimulate the prostate. This is known as the million-dollar point.

6. The frenulum, located on the underside of the head of the penis, is a fantastic stimulation point, a sort of male clitoris. A man can have a blended orgasm if the prostate and the frenulum are stimulated simultaneously! Women, you can greatly please a man by stroking this area with your thumbs. If you stroke his frenulum with one thumb and his testes up from the bottom with your other thumb, he will be a very happy man. If he gets aroused too quickly, stop stroking the frenulum and gently press in at the base of the penis, just above the testes, with your other thumb. Gentle testes-tickling while stroking (or not stroking) is something we men just love.

A man has to become something of a gynecologist and a woman a proctologist if they want to increase each other's orgasmic potential. I know: If you're a women, you're thinking, "I put up with enough of his s$%t, now I have to probe it?" And if you're a guy, you're thinking, "Oh, no, she's not putting anything up there!" But sooner or later, you're going to have to go to the doc to get that exam. At least this one is more enjoyable, with significantly happier results.

G-SPOT MASSAGE AND FEMALE EJACULATION

Did you know that, for some women who haven't experienced a G-spot orgasm, the reason is that the "spot" has not yet been sensitized? Believe it or not, the G-spot, like a muscle, sometimes has to be activated and worked out in order to work up to an orgasm. In my experience, many women who say they haven't had an internal orgasm claim the G-spot doesn't really exist, they don't have one, or, worse, that something is wrong with them. Others say they don't feel worthy or it's immoral. Altogether, these add up to some very sensitive and often painful issues for many women.

Although a woman can and will try to help you find her G-spot, I feel it is a man's job to relieve her from having to concern herself too much. Let her tell you where, like scratching an itch, she needs to feel you until you both learn her spots. Communicate! Remember, women have both left and right sides of their brain firing all the time. You want to keep her amygdala (worry center) out of the sex equation as much as possible.

If you are a man fortunate, yes, fortunate enough to be the one who can guide and accompany a woman through any one of these situations—be glad. It takes work and skill, and even if it doesn't work right away, it will enable you both to grow in ways not possible with a typical relationship. Sometimes orgasms happen by happy accident of a good fit. If people are fortunate to have such a fit, great! But a good physical fit does not a relationship make. Good relating makes a good relationship, and understanding and discovery are far more important than a good physical fit will ever be. It is through the process of understanding, discovery, and communication that you will most likely go on to find and create new ways to achieve orgasm.

Remember, all thoughts of "performance" must go. Performance can only be considered after the right spots have been found or coaxed into being. A great way to bring them into play is to do just that: play, with no expectations. Then it becomes a matter of patience, passion, precision, and perseverance.

The G-spot, like the AFE and PFE, is just a bundle of nerves. When Dr. Mehmet Oz was asked by Joy Behar about the existence of the often elusive G-spot, he replied, "Considering science has proven we all begin life as female, and the male prostate is stimulated by the same nerves that stimulate the G-spot, it is not possible that those nerves just disappear." I have personal experience with girlfriends who thought they didn't have a G-spot, but, like a credit card, that G-spot just need to be activated to work!

Once you have established where your partner's G-spot is, make sure she has emptied her bladder and you have ample lubrication.

G-SPOT MASSAGE

1. Have your lover lie on the bed.
2. Kneel on her right side and place your left hand slightly above her pubic bone.
3. *Make eye contact.* She must be made to feel completely comfortable.
4. Gently introduce your well-lubricated hand to her vulva and vaginal area.
5. Begin gently rubbing and massaging with sweeping, up-and-down and circular motions. This should last for several minutes, with constant reassuring eye contact. Talk with her: Ask how it feels and whether she is ready to be entered.
6. Position your fingers up and inside her as if holding a bowling ball.
7. Gently find her G-spot with your two inside fingers (fig. 36, page 247).
8. Once you do, begin gently pressing down above her pubic bone with your left hand. Gently begin your massage, pressing upward in a back-and-forth, come-hither motion across the G-spot. This movement should emanate from your elbow, moving forward and backward using your shoulder as a hinge.
9. Begin slowly, then gradually speed up according to her response and needs. It is also good to practice curling your finger back and forth at various speeds.
10. Try using the palm of your hand to maintain friction on the clitoris while you're stimulating the G-spot.

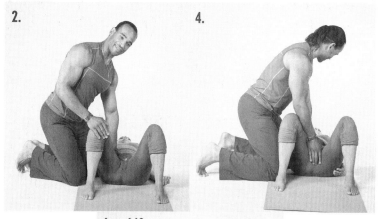

2.

4.

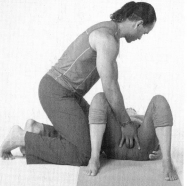

6. and 10.

For years, *Cosmopolitan* has been providing sex tips for women on how to please a man. By writing this book, I'm just trying to create balance in the bedroom.

If she wishes to climax . . .

1. If she sounds like she is about to reach a climactic point (listen to her breathing), ask her if she wants to.
2. If she does, press down deeper with your left hand and move your right hand more vigorously.
3. Continue using the palm of your hand to maintain friction on the clitoris while you are stimulating the G-spot.
4. Once she starts, do not stop until she says, "Stop!"

If she wants to (and is able to) ejaculate . . .

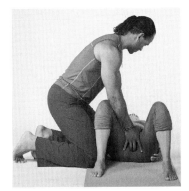

1. Continue using your two fingers to pull in a deliberate yet gentle upward and outward motion. Do not switch positions or styles if she starts breathing more quickly and deeply. As she is releasing, begin a deeper, more vigorous right-hand triggering motion.
2. Even though she may feel as though she is going to urinate, have her push through her core, and voilà!
3. As she begins to ejaculate, move your palm away from her clitoris and begin more of an outward pulling motion to allow for the ejaculate to flow unobstructed.
4. Do not stop until she says, "Stop!"

MANUAL AFE STIMULATION

Here you are using the middle finger to stimulate the AFE. What you want to do first is prepare her for entry. Do not ever just try to put your finger inside her without allowing her to relax first. I'm not saying she should not be aroused; she should. You also want to make sure she is well lubricated. Try a pelvic massage first. After you have spent five to ten minutes on pelvic massage, including clitoral stimulation, slowly work your finger in and gently ease it back to her AFE. You will feel it at the upper rear at the base of her cervix. Slowly and gently begin pushing up, drawing small circles and then pulling back with a short "come hither" motion. You want to press a little stronger as you go along, but watch her face, body, and breathing. You can progressively speed up your pressing and pulling back as she feels more comfortable, again watching and listening. Continue until she has an orgasm or is about to. If you wish to build up energy for a stronger orgasm, wait a while; do not overstimulate her right then. You can also gently simultaneously stimulate her clitoris with your other hand.

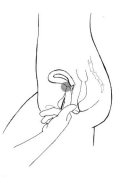

fig. 38

Turn off the TV. Go to bed early. Stay up late. I would say bring extra napkins, but if all goes well, a towel will be more appropriate.

BREATHING ROOM

One way for partners to establish a more intimate connection is to practice breathing together. The Yab Yum Straddle is a good example of how breathing together can help establish the deep trust and intimacy needed for a couple to open up to each other. Sitting together, simply breathing and becoming each other's breath, can make this happen, and it's simply beautiful. While she breathes out, he breathes in, and vice versa. Try this sitting on the floor; on pillows; on the bed; even lying facing each other, pressed together, feeling each other's bellies complement your inhale and exhale. Talk about close!

Another form of breathing that is important to learn is breathing during sex. For example, during the Hip Drop, practice exhaling as you're dropping so you can prolong your intimacy by staving off the orgasm until you're ready. You are drawing in energy on the inhalation, breathing it down the front of your body, and exhaling on the Hip Drop, pumping the energy up the spine. This will help sustain energy throughout your lovemaking. You should also notice, as you practice prolonging coitus, that it is not the man who falls asleep after orgasm but the woman. Successful sex has the opposite effect of typical sex, where the man falls asleep afterward.

PREPARE HER FOR PLEASURE

A woman's greatest desire is to be desired, so a man must make her feel wanted! Aside from that, you must create an ambience and set a mood to prepare a woman for pleasure. Even a quickie is the result of preparation. Intimacy with a woman is *never* an isolated event. If you want loving all night long, you have to prepare her all day long. Intimacy with a woman is more like preparing a Thanksgiving dinner than barbecuing. I know most guys just want to be grillin' and chillin' as soon as possible, but you still have to wait for the coals to start glowing before you can get going, right?

A sweet evening should start with sweet words during the day, gestures to make her feel acknowledged and wanted. Remember the old saying, "A man needs sex to feel good but a woman needs to feel good to have sex?" If you're at home and you want to make love after dinner, then you make dinner, or at least do the dishes. The longer it takes her to wind down, the longer it will take her to warm up. While the dishes are soaking in the sink, she should be soaking in the bathtub by candlelight. When she gets out of the tub, greet her with a warm towel and some warm lotion or oil.

Sex should not be an occurrence but an event. The less she has to think or plan, the more she'll treat you like a man.

A woman's orgasm is in need of special circumstances, a marriage of arousal and relaxation. If a man can't arouse *and* relax her, he can't climax her. To do this you must allow her to enter something of a Zen Zone. People think of Zen as a state of perfect calm only, but it is actually a perfectly balanced calm in the midst of other things. As in all things Zen, it is important to stay present. Remember that sex is a marathon, not a sprint, and orgasm, especially for a woman, is only one point on a continuum. Sex is not a linear event unless you are in an early stage of understanding it. You want to stay in the zone throughout the encounter.

Guys, I don't know how else to say it: You need to work to become what you want to attract. If you want a lover who is in shape, you need to lay off the six-pack you buy and work on the six-pack you build.

Sometimes talking about sex is harder than doing it. Use this book as a way to talk to each other. You might be amazed by what you find.

PREPARE HIM FOR PLEASURE

Preparing a man for pleasure is simple: Be nice to him. Do not emasculate him. Do not put him down. If you take away his spine and his balls, you will limit his lovemaking abilities! Appreciate what he is trying to do for you and your relationship. A man wants to feel respected and appreciated for his efforts, for what he *wants* to do for you. If lovers both take care of each other outside the bedroom they will take better care of each other inside the bedroom. It works both ways. Men really do want to please their lovers. It is our greatest, deepest desire—so tell us what you like. Guide us. We are task-oriented.

We also enjoy a massage just as much as women do. The perineum massage works especially well for us, even if it is not the internal prostate massage. It makes a big difference in how we feel at the point of orgasm.

Reciprocate! The more we do for each other, the more we will want to do for each other. Remember, we all want to feel good about ourselves, and we all want to feel wanted.

That being said . . . ladies, keep up your figure. You can either have dessert or be dessert. I'm not talking about being thin; I'm talking about being in good physical shape for your body type. Thin does not necessarily mean healthy, and "not fat" does not mean "in shape." Men like cushion for the pushin', and junk in the trunk is appreciated. Whoever said that the way to a man's heart is through his stomach flunked geography! Create a hunger in him for you. A man's biggest turn-on is a woman who desires him; dare I say, that's most of the allure of porn stars and strippers. The Madonna/whore complex is a man's main fantasy, like the stereotypical secretary with glasses and her hair up. Both men and women love paradox. We want a balance of both naughty and nice.

Men are visual, so the soccer-mom sweat-suit thing doesn't work for us any more than unshowered, unshaven, and unemployed works for women. A man wants to know what he's working for. He doesn't mind going to work if he's got someone special to come home to. Greet him with a hero's welcome at the door when he comes home from battle, and he'll rock you like a Viking in heat. If he's reading this book, he's already on his way to having the skills to thrill you.

Though this book can provide exercises and skills to become a better lover, there is no substitute for the realization of love within yourself. Before you can truly be fit for love or find someone who's a perfect fit, you must be a better lover yourself. You can only give what you have. Learning to love yourself is the ultimate orgasm.

MONOGAMY DOES NOT MEAN MONOTONY

*b*EING FIT FOR LOVE is not just being better in bed. It's being better in every area of your life—your relationships in and out of the bedroom, your work, your daily interactions with friends and family. Everything you do ultimately plays a part in your love life. If you are struggling to get along with people in general, your relationship with your lover may also suffer. Are you drinking, drugging, gambling, or carousing? Whatever you are acting out in your life will come home to bed with you sooner or later.

When people ask me about the importance of working out, they usually expect me to comment on physical training. They ask how I stay in such great shape at forty-four years old. I say, first of all, that I practice what I preach—a mind-set and way of being—and the body follows. I tell them I train my spirit and my brain while I train my body, that for every hour I'm in the gym I spend three hours in study, meditation, and contemplation. I tell them that I take more vitamins for my brain than I do for my body, and spend far more time looking into how I act than how I look. I tell them that although I take care of my outside, that sex is truly an inside job. I tell them that I continue to work to become what I hope to attract, and that I give my lover what I ask from her in return: my best!

When guys ask me how they can become better lovers, I tell them not to be selfish, to learn and remember what their lover likes and adapt to their lover's needs, to work through the inevitable ups and downs of a relationship. To be mentally fit for love, you have to train yourself to be good at all of these things—to *become what you hope to attract.*

To be emotionally fit for love, you must watch for times when you are upset or disappointed with your lover. Occasionally your partner will, like you, make a mistake. Be sure to pick your battles wisely; make sure that what you bring up is worth talking about, and address issues that concern you in a compassionate and non-confrontational way. If they do something that upsets or concerns you, try saying something like, "When you said or did this or that, it really bothered, hurt, worried, or concerned me. Why did you say or do that?" If you don't feel you can talk openly with your partner, you might not be with the right person; or perhaps you are both afraid of what the other person might think, or even of meeting your true self. Be brave! The easier it is for you to relate to your lover out of bed, the easier it will be for you to relate in bed. Communication is key to copulation. Remember, you are in any relationship to grow, especially through difficulty. You are not in a relationship to control the other person. If you want to be a better lover, seek first to understand then to be understood.

I have been far from perfect in this regard. Because I worked as a stripper, I had trained myself to be an immature idiot when it came to women. Anytime I saw something I didn't like in the woman I was with, I left. Hey, it wasn't like there was a shortage of opportunity, right? I thought I was seeing something that I didn't like about them, but what I've learned is that I really saw something I didn't like about myself. In the gym, or in a dance class, you look regularly into a mirror to check your form. In a relationship, your lover is your mirror. Before you consider rubbing up against their naked body, consider that if the relationship is worth anything, you will also rub up against your own issues and insecurities. If you are wise, you will be glad: You will face your fear and grow. Remember, you can't go together if you don't grow together. Growing together builds trust and intimacy. A great relationship is like an alchemical fire. It can expose and turn your burdens into blessings if you let it.

Being fit for love is about becoming physically, mentally, spiritually, and emotionally ready for an intimate relationship. You will have better moves, a better body, and most importantly a love connection with more depth, passion, and understanding of your lover and yourself than you ever believed possible. So I encourage you to build your body, train your mind, and feed your soul. By doing so, you will become—and therefore attract—an amazing lover.

Monogamy means monotony to many, but it does not have to. Often, when we are looking to break free from what we perceive to be a boring situation, what we are looking for is not someone else but something else to change the way we feel. When I was first learning to meditate, my teacher asked me if I was bored, and I said yes. He told me that the problem was not that I was bored, but that I was boring. We need to learn to see any and all situations with new eyes. Wayne Dyer says, "When you change the way you look at things, the things you look at change." This applies to people, too, who are always changing whether we are awake enough to notice or not. So the question becomes: Are we willing to not only become what we want to attract but also keep what we want?

Once you know how to go deeper with someone, both physically and emotionally, you have the foundation to experience each other and yourself in a whole new way. I've said it before: You can't expect to find oil if you dig shallow holes. So find one and dig deep—dig very deep. Dig a ravine, look in, and keep looking. Then as Nietzsche says, "If you look deep enough into that ravine, the ravine begins to look into you!" The more you look into the mirror, the more it looks into you because it allows you to see yourself more clearly. A good lover, like a good mirror, helps you to love yourself. In a Rumi poem, a lover was asked, "Do you love me more than you love yourself"? The reply was, "I love you, I love myself, I love myself, I love you!" I laugh at what I thought was sex or even sexy before I really learned this. Once you go deep enough into each other, into sex, you will find the highest of highs there. You will find God (if you need to substitute this with the Divine or Heaven or Higher Self, please do!), and you will find God within your Lover. When you are able to find God within and through your lover, you are truly Fit for Love!

ACKNOWLEDGMENTS

MY GRATITUDE AND THANKS go out to the following people who helped make this book possible.

To my friend and editor Wendy Merrill, not only for the wonderful job she did in such a short time on this book, but for believing in me and my work to begin with. I highly recommend her book, *Falling into Manholes: The Memoir of a Bad/Good Girl*, to anybody who wants a humorous, scary, experiential peek into what happens in a woman's head and heart when she gets lost in intimate relationships.

Thank you to Matthew Lore and everyone at The Experiment for taking a chance on me as a first-time author and giving me an opportunity to share my work. And thank you to Christine Cipriani for her query-intensive editing, which not only made the book better but also made me a better writer.

Peter Ivory, my friend, photographer, and videographer for putting his equipment in harm's way to photograph me. He is talented, wise, and brave.

Bonnie Neer for her artwork and diagrams, as well as her friendship and support throughout this process. Bonnie and her girls, Gretchen and Caroline, have seen me through so much, as well as helping me with my Web site.

Ahna Fender for her editorial and spiritual input.

Bruce Stevens for his friendship, insight, and support while I was getting myself established in the Bay Area. He not only put me up; he put up with me.

Dr. Khanti Patel for his mentorship and friendship during my years of research and questioning.

Bruce Goldstein for his support during my time in Florida.

Dr. Terri Larsen, a great friend and healer.

Vince LaQuaglia, my friend and first mentor.

Taylor, often my greatest teacher, for modeling in this book and being there to witness many of my most profound life lessons and breakthroughs. I thank her for her support and belief in me.

To all spiritual teachers, healers, scientists, medical, health-care, and fitness professionals and all psychological, emotional, and sexual-health workers past and present, for we are all in this together.

Also, to the women I have been in relationships with, thank you for putting up with me and my foolishness and stupidity during my growth stages. You have taught me much.

In memory of my parents and my brother, Scott, I would like to give thanks for the gift of their time, love, and lessons. I thank my sister Robyn for taking me fishing at 5 a.m. and teaching me to drive in the cemetery where I couldn't kill anyone, and both Robyn and my sister Nikki for putting up with me and my often overly introspective, then overtly expressive antics. I love and appreciate all of you.

And finally, thank you, readers for your interest in this work, and in this play.

INDEX

Leg (or Two) Ups, 222–24
lesbians, xiii, 31
Love Locks
    Cervix, 15, 62–63
    Lumbar, 13, 15, 38–40, 69–70,
        74–75, 104–15, 132–33, 136–43
    overview, 7–11, 16, 19
    Sacral/Coccyx, 12, 64–65, 242
    Thoracic, 14, 15, 36–37, 44–46,
        136–37
lover undercover, xii
loving yourself, 259, 263
Lumbar Love Lock, 13, 15, 38–40,
        69–70, 74–75, 104–15,
        132–33, 136–43
lumbar region, 7–9, 15
lumbar stretches, 38–40, 47, 58

male hot spots, 24–25
male orgasms, 30–31
marriage and sex, 191
Mars, Billy Sunday, ix–xii
martial arts movements, 154–55,
        163–72, 174–87
massage, 73, 238–55
Mayas, 158–60
Mencia, Carlos, 24
Milkshake, The, 234
mirroring, 194–95, 197
Missionary Positions, 162, 198,
        199, 200, 206–7
Modified Cobra Abdominal
        Stretch, 46
Modified Pigeons, 47, 72–73
monogamy, xiii, 261–64
movement
    importance of, x–xi, 163
    matching sex positions and,
        198–212

overview, xii–xiii
pain and/or injuries, 41
See also exercises; stretches

Naughty Kneeling Ninjas, 170–72,
        174–77, 180–85
Neck and Shoulders Stretch, 62–63
Nietzsche, 264

occipital and sacral massage,
        239–40
Oprah, 191, 194
orgasms
    female orgasms, 27–30, 199–
        200, 219
    hormones released during, 22
    and Kundalini energy, 2–3
    male orgasms, 30–31
    overview, 26–27
    spine and, 6, 27, 30–31, 32, 44

parasympathetic nervous system,
        19, 22
partner-assisted stretching, 68–85
Pelvic Massage, 242, 244–49
pelvic nerve, 20–21
Pelvic Perineum Stretch, 64–65,
        126–27
pelvis and pelvic tilts, 10–11
Pendulum, The, 4, 161, 180–81
Perineal Massage, 242, 244–49
perineum (pelvic floor), 20, 31, 32,
        64, 126–27, 128, 244, 258
PFE (Posterior Fornix Erogenous)
        zone, 24, 27, 200, 201, 204,
        208, 210
phenomenal sex, 18
physical attractiveness ratio, 10
Pin-down Doll, 201, 217

ABOUT THE AUTHOR

BILLY SUNDAY MARS, orphaned as a teen, dove into boxing, Eastern philosophy, and dance in his search for love, purpose, and spiritual fulfillment. As an athlete, artist, and spiritual seeker, he became an erotic dancer and instructor in Japan and China, where he also studied martial arts and massage. After moving back to the United States, he studied Tantric disciplines and worked as a fitness trainer. Now a sought-after "Romantic Fitness" expert, Billy has combined his understanding of sexuality and fitness into his proprietary Fit for Love program. He teaches Fit for Love and related classes in San Francisco and in Marin County, California, where he lives.